Notice

This book has been withdrawn from health library stock for one or more of the following reasons:

- There is a more recent edition of the title
- The book is more than 10 years old and more current material on the topic is available

You are therefore strongly advised to check any information contained within this book before using it to inform patient care

Seromyotomy for Chronic Duodenal Ulcer

General Editor, Wolfe Surgical Atlases:
William F. Walker, DSc, ChM, FRCS (Edin. and England), FRS (Edin.).

Single Surgical Procedures 10

A Colour Atlas of

Seromyotomy for Chronic Duodenal Ulcer

T. Vincent Taylor
MD, ChM, FRCS, FRCSE
Consultant Surgical Gastroenterologist, Manchester Royal Infirmary, Lecturer in Surgery, University of Manchester. Previously Hunterian Professor Royal College of Surgeons of England and Moynihan Medallist.

(Photography by University Department of Medical Illustration, Manchester Royal Infirmary)

Wolfe Medical Publications Ltd

Published by Wolfe Medical Publications Ltd, 1984
Printed by Royal Smeets Offset b.v., Weert, Netherlands
ISBN 0 7234 1013 5

This book is one of the titles in the series of Wolfe Single Surgical Procedures, a series which will eventually cover some 200 titles.

If you wish to be kept informed of new additions to the series and receive details of our other titles, please write to Wolfe Medical Publications Ltd, Wolfe House, 3 Conway Street, London W1P 6HE.

A few of the other titles in print and in preparation in the Single Surgical Procedures series

Parotidectomy
Traditional Meniscectomy
Inguinal Hernias & Hydroceles in Infants and Children
Surgery for Pancreatic & Associated Carcinomata
Subtotal Thyroidectomy
Boari Bladder-Flap Procedure
Treatment of Carpal Tunnel Syndrome
Anterior Resection of Rectum
Seromyotomy for Chronic Duodenal Ulcer
Resection of Aortic Aneurysm
Modified Radical Mastectomy
Total Gastrectomy
Ileo-Rectal Anastomosis
Pre-Prosthetic Oral Surgery
Surgery for Undescended Testes
Techniques of Nerve Grafting and Repair
Surgery for Dupuytren's Contracture
Athrodesis of the Ankle
Surgery for Congenital Dislocation of the Hip
Common Operations of the Foot
Femoral and Tibial Osteotomy
Maxillo-Facial Traumatology
Surgery for Chondromalacia Patellae
Stabilisation for Extensive Spinal Injury
Spondylolisthesis
Laminectomy
Gall Bladder Cholecystectomy
Repair of Prolapsed Rectum
Proctocolectomy
Resection of Oesophagus
Splenectomy
Thyroid Lobectomy
Hirschprung's Disease
Extra-cranial and Intra-cranial Anastomosis
Anterior Nephrectomy
Bladder Augmentation
Caecocystoplasty
Hiatus Hernia
Total Gastrectomy
Billroth 1 Gastrectomy
Billroth 2 Gastrectomy
Abdominal Incisions
Thoracotomy
Chronic Pancreatitis Operation
Surgery for Strictures in Common Bile Duct
Biliary Enteric Anastomosis
Partial Hepatectomy
Splenectomy
Right Hemicolectomy
Appendicectomy
Incisional Hernia
Lung Lobectomy
Lung Removal
Gastric Reconstruction
Surgery for Lymphoedema
Kidney Transplants
Liver Transplant
Pancreas Transplant
Dialysis Techniques
Surgery for Thoracic Outlet
Haemorrhoids
Abdominoperineal Resection of Rectum
Rectosigmoid Resection
Non-resectional Surgery for Multiple Bowel Stenosis
Surgery for Anorectal Incontinence
Carotid Surgery
Craniotomy
Parathyroidectomy
Arterial Injuries
Arterial Bypass Grafts in Leg
Visceral Vascular Occlusion
Varicose Veins under Local Anaesthesia
Aortofemoral Bypass
Aortoilac Disobliteration
Technique of Small Vessel Repair
Technique of Nerve Grafting and Repair
Microsurgery Techniques
Reimplantation of Ureters
Pyloric Stenosis in Children
Cleft Palate
Anorectal Malformation
Amputations of the Lower Limb
Anterolateral Decompression
Spinal Fusion
Scoliosis
Spinal Fusion for Low Back Pain
Anterior Fusion of Cervical Spine
Recurrent Dislocation of Shoulder
Joint Replacement of Elbow
Joint Replacement of Wrist and Hand
Operative Fixation of Fractures of the Forearm
Joint Replacement at the Hip
Joint Replacement at the Knee
Arthrodesis of the Knee
Triple Arthrodesis
Discogram Surgery – Lumbar Disc
Amputations of the Upper Limb and Hand
Plastering Techniques
Operations for Peripheral Nerve
Compression Syndromes
Techniques of Tendon Transfer in the Upper Limb
Arthrodesis of the Wrist
Reconstructive Procedures of the Thumb
Flexor Tendon Repair and Grafting
Minor Operative Procedures
Technique of Arthroscopy of the Knee
Management of Fresh Ligamentous Injuries of the Knee
Technique of Complete Denture Construction
Partial Denture Design
Wisdom Tooth Surgery
Apicectomy
Surgery of the Temporomandibular Joint
Dental Occlusion
Periodontology
Pre-prosthetic Oral Surgery
Endodontics Surgery

Contents

Acknowledgements

I am grateful to Mr G. Rogers, Head of the Medical Illustration Department and his staff for the photography, and to Mrs J. Mathias for typing the text.

Introduction

Peptic ulcer surgery became feasible after the first successful gastrectomy and gastroenterostomy, which were performed by Billroth and Wölfler respectively in 1881.

The turn of the century coincided with a marked increase in the prevalence of duodenal ulcer. This century has produced four eras, during which fundamental changes of attitude have occurred. The era of gastroenterostomy, in view of the high incidence of recurrent ulcer, gave way to Polya gastrectomy. The increased mortality, post-gastrectomy syndromes, and long-term nutritional sequelae next led surgeons to use the newly developing vagotomy. Truncal vagotomy and drainage is complicated by distension (50 per cent), dumping (25 per cent), and diarrhoea (30 per cent), as a result of which the era of the pylorus-preserving operations has been entered.

Highly selective vagotomy embodies the sound physiological principles of parietal-cell vagotomy with pylorus preservation. Dumping and diarrhoea are virtually abolished, but the operation may be technically difficult and tedious to perform; also, in some series, recurrence rates of over 20 per cent have been recorded, while in others rates are 5 per cent or less at five years. These high rates of ulcer recurrence have been consequent upon incomplete and inadequate denervation of the parietal-cell mass as a result of technical difficulties.

Anterior lesser curve seromyotomy with posterior truncal vagotomy has been developed as a pylorus-preserving operation in which the parietal-cell mass is denervated, but which is technically safe, simple, and speedily performed.

Indications for surgery

The major indications for elective duodenal ulcer surgery are: chronicity, failed medical treatment, frequent early relapse after cessation of medical treatment or maintenance therapy, and repeated gastrointestinal tract haemorrhage. The operation may be performed as an emergency procedure when bleeding is present. The ulcer is then oversewn through a duodenotomy and the pylorus may be preserved.

Contraindications

The major contraindication to this operation is pyloric stenosis, when anterior seromyotomy and posterior truncal vagotomy may be carried out, but a drainage procedure is then required. Dilatation of the pylorus is probably inadequate for the patient with well-established pyloric stenosis. The coincidental performance of a cholecystectomy is not a contraindication to this operation, as preservation both of the hepatic branches of the anterior vagus and of the pylorus appears to prevent the high incidence of diarrhoea and bile reflux gastritis which complicate truncal vagotomy, drainage, and cholecystectomy.

Preoperative preparation

Little specific preoperative preparation is required other than that used routinely for an elective abdominal operation. A nasogastric tube is passed after induction of anaesthesia and intravenous fluids are given.

Complications

Over 350 of these operations have now been performed. There have been no deaths and no immediate complications directly attributable to the gastric surgery. In the early postoperative period a small number of cases have developed delayed gastric emptying which has persisted in one per cent, these requiring a drainage procedure. Gastric emptying studies have been performed and with the exception of slightly accelerated early emptying of liquids, these rates are normal. Occasional wound infections have occurred. As a prophylaxis against these infections I now inject a broad-spectrum antibiotic, such as cephamandole 1g or mezlocillin 2g diluted in 10 ml of water, into the wound as anaesthesia is induced (pre-incisional administration).

In patients over 50 years of age, intravenous low molecular weight dextran or subcutaneous heparin are valuable aids as prophylaxis against deep-venous thrombosis.

Results

In my personal series of 96 of these operations performed over a four-year period, I have had one proven ulcer recurrence in the pre-pyloric region of the stomach. I am aware of an additional two recurrences which have occurred in patients of my colleagues. Only with a complete five-year to ten-year follow-up will an accurate assessment of recurrence be possible.

Most recurrent ulcers after vagotomy, however, occur within one year; moreover, I believe that as anterior lesser curve seromyotomy with posterior truncal vagotomy represents a greater degree of gastric vagal denervation than highly selective vagotomy, the rates of recurrence are more likely to approximate to those encountered after truncal vagotomy (five per cent) than to some of the unsatisfactory results that have been reported by some surgeons after conventional highly selective vagotomy.

Expedients of peptic ulcer surgery

The expedients of peptic ulcer surgery are:

1 The parietal-cell mass should be completely denervated;
2 The pylorus should be preserved;
3 Gastric emptying should be near normal;
4 The loss of adaptive relaxation inherent in denervation of the proximal stomach should, at least in part, be compensated for;
5 Duodenogastric reflux must be minimised;
6 The incidence of distension, dumping and diarrhoea should be low;
7 The operation must be safe, simple and rapidly performed;
8 The risks of damage to the nerve of Latarjet and of ischaemic necrosis must be overcome;
9 The incidence of recurrent ulcer must be acceptably low: vagotomy must be as complete as is permissible to preserve normal gastric emptying.

It is with these aims in view that anterior lesser curve seromyotomy with posterior truncal vagotomy has been devised, investigated and developed.

Preparation and incision

1a

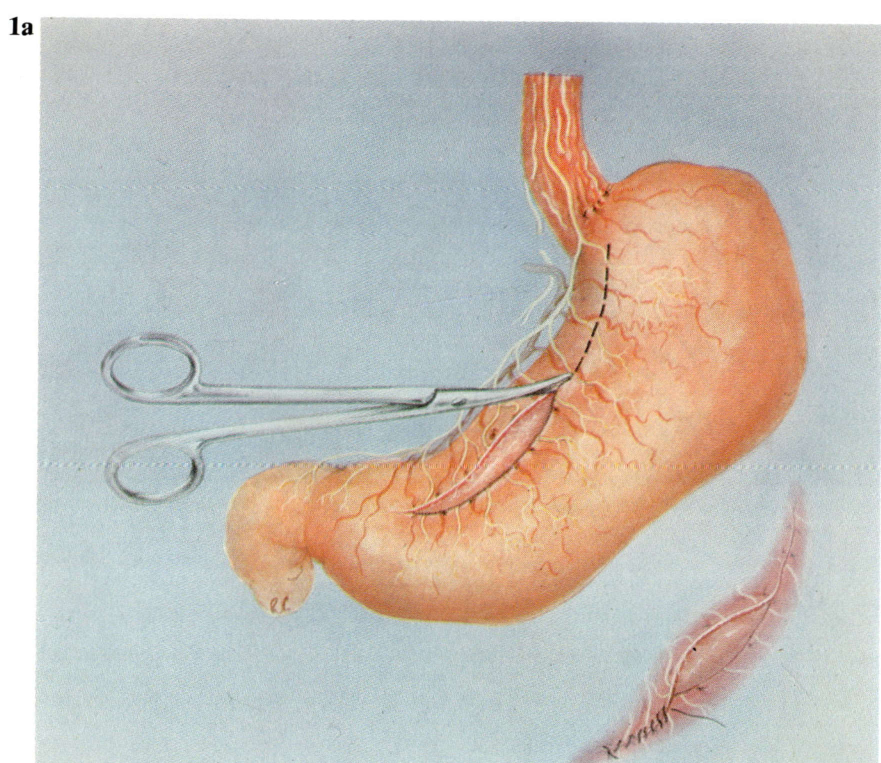

1a **Diagrammatic representation of anterior lesser curve seromyotomy with posterior truncal vagotomy.**

1b

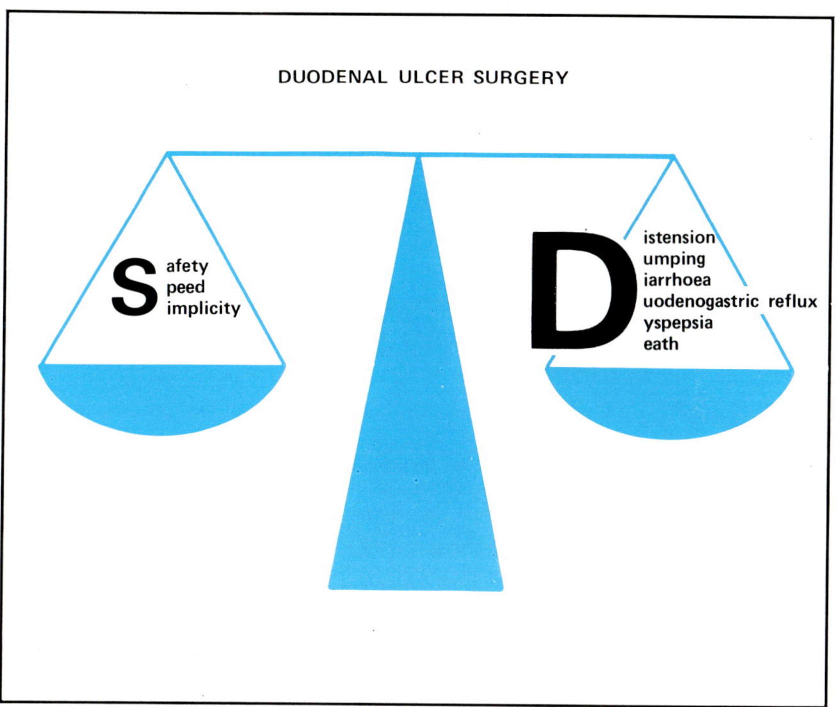

1b Balance in surgery. The balance in peptic ulcer surgery oscillates between, on the one hand the expedients – safety, speed and simplicity and, on the other the disadvantages of dumping, diarrhoea, distension, duodenogastric reflux, recurrent dyspepsia, and death. More conservative procedures have on the whole been associated with higher rates of recurrence, while the more radical operations have higher morbidity and mortality.

2 The patient is anaesthetised and placed supine on the operating table, the whole abdomen being exposed.

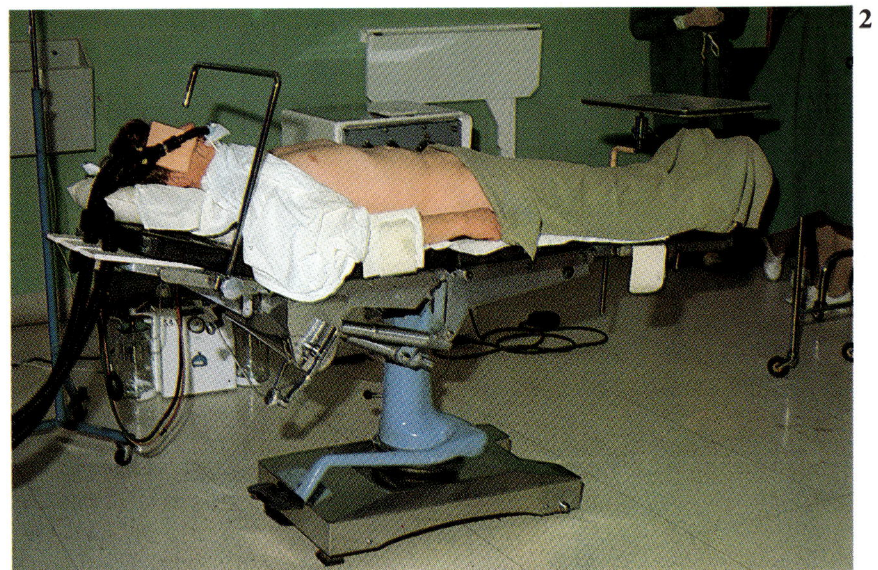

2

3 The anterior abdominal wall is painted with an antiseptic skin preparation, such as povidone iodine, between the line of the nipples and the pubic symphysis, extending laterally as far as the mid-clavicular lines.

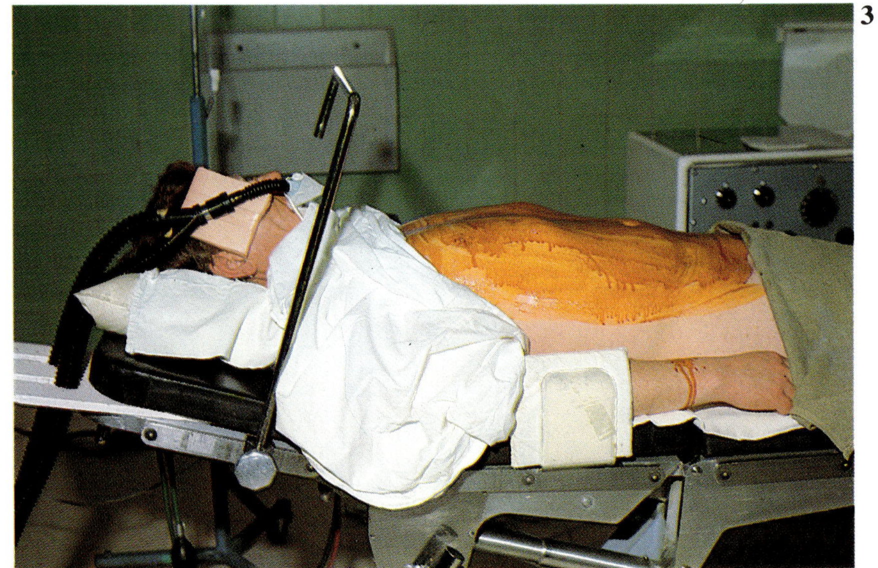

3

4 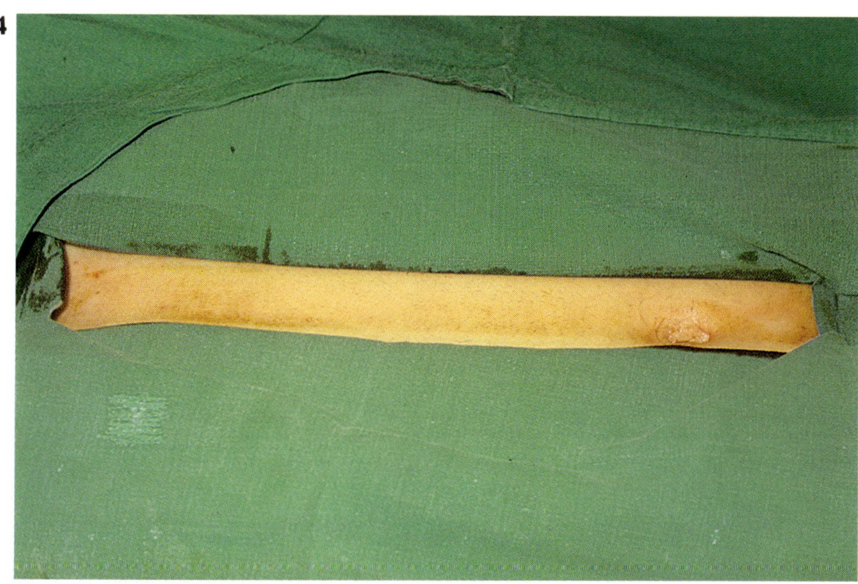

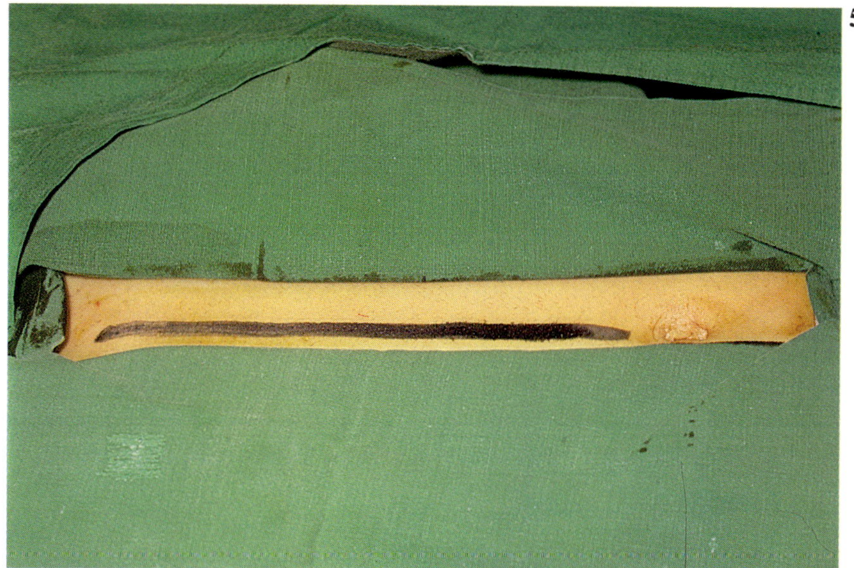 5

4 The towels are placed in preparation for an upper midline incision.

5 The incision extends from the xiphoid process of the sternum to the superior aspect of the umbilicus.

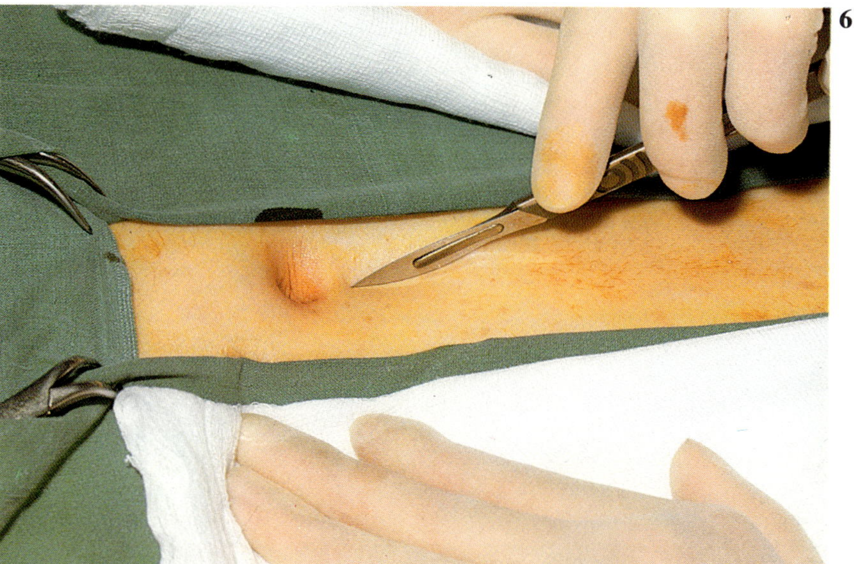 6

6 Use of antibiotic. It is my practice to infiltrate the tissue behind the incision with a broad-spectrum antibiotic such as cephamandole (1g) diluted with 10 ml of water. This is introduced by a spinal needle as the patient is anaesthetised, using a single puncture site. The skin incision is then carried out.

7 The skin incision is deepened down to the linea alba.

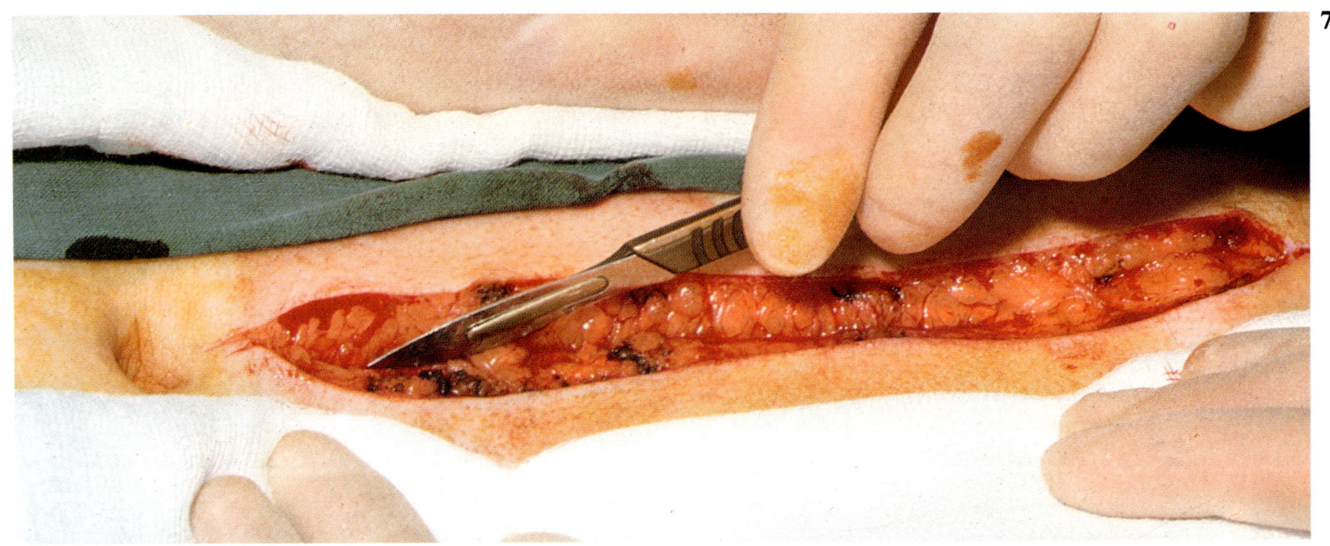

7

8 Haemostasis is secured.

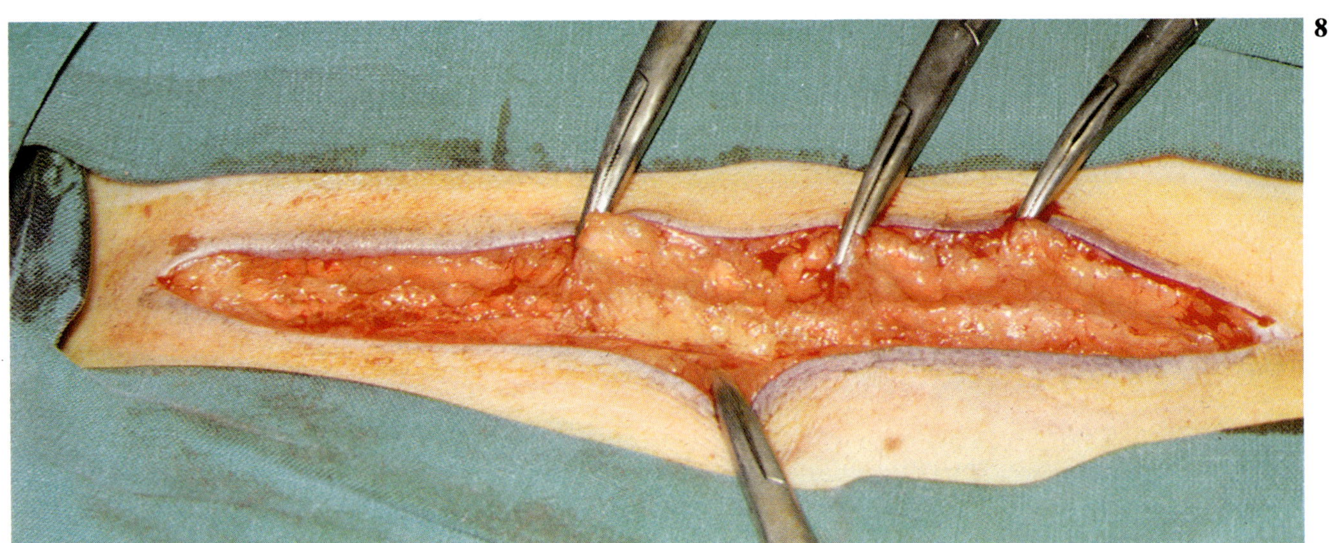

8

9 The linea alba is incised.

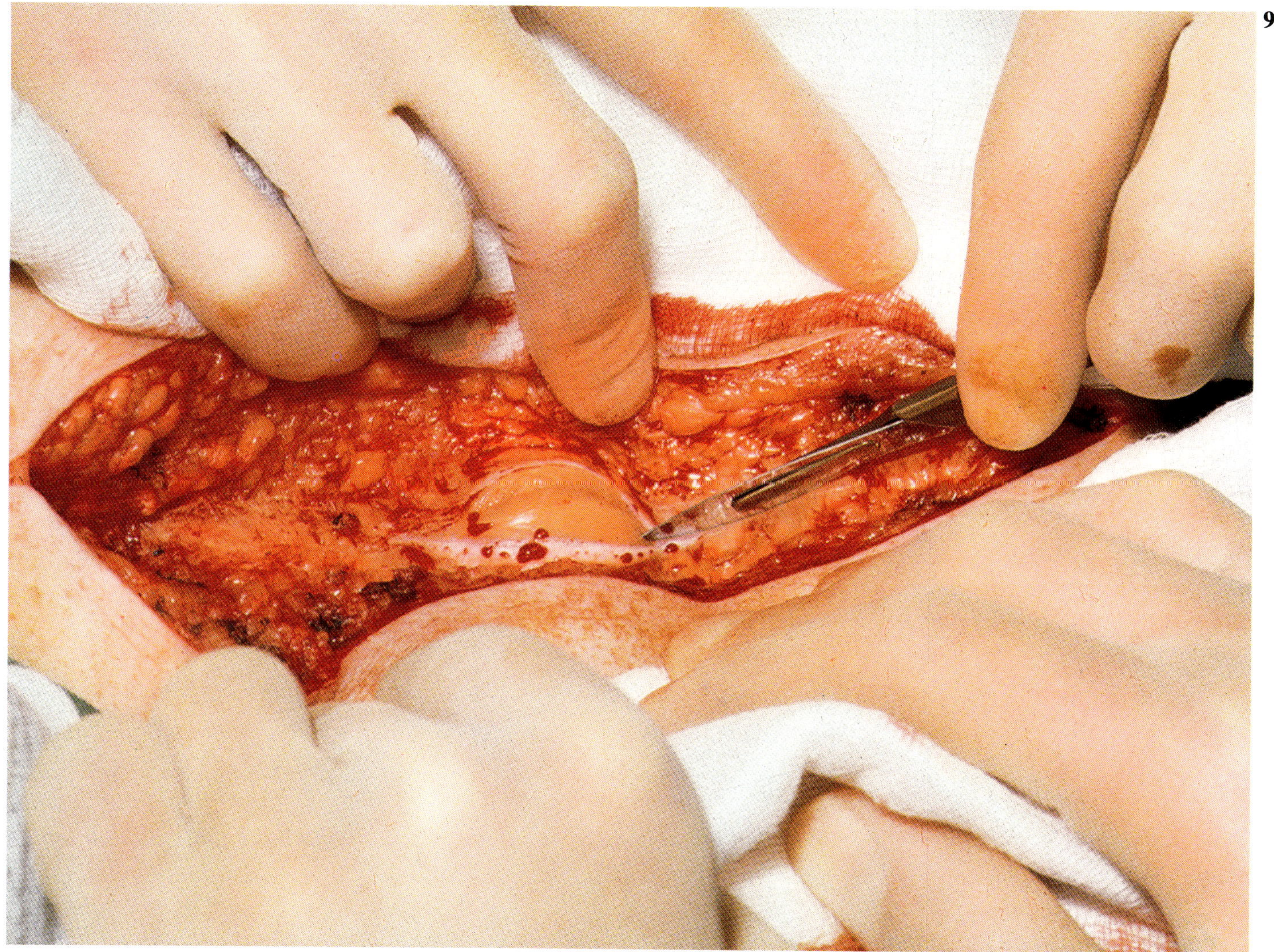
9

10 The peritoneal fat is exposed.

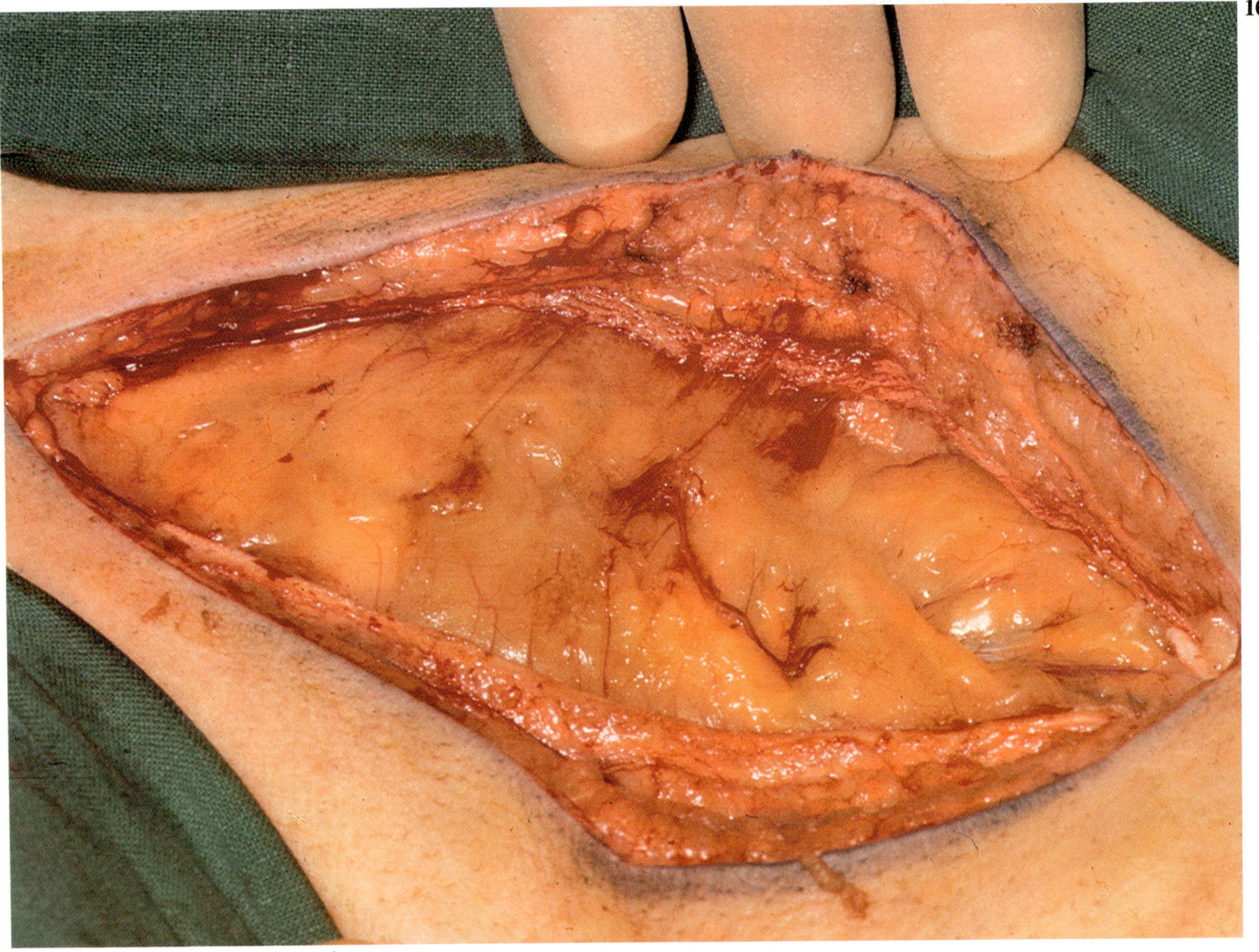

10

11

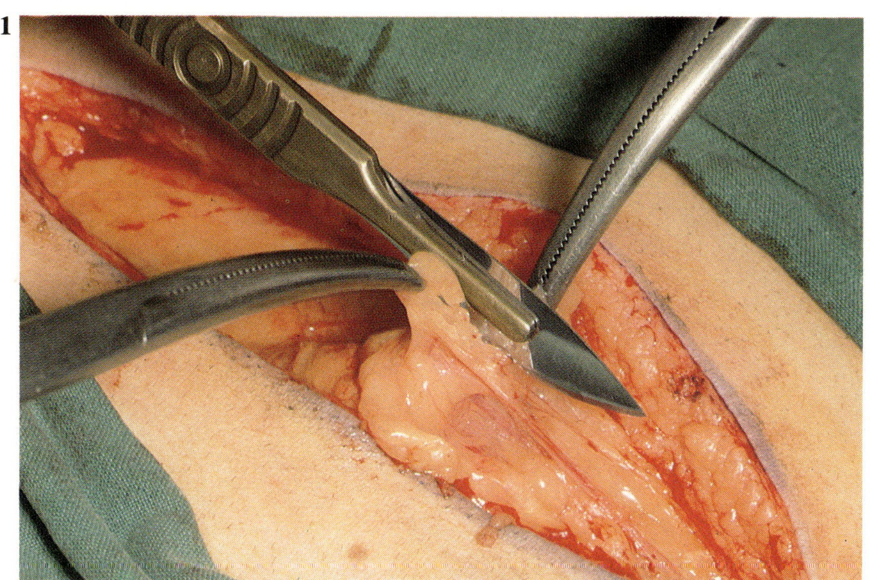

12

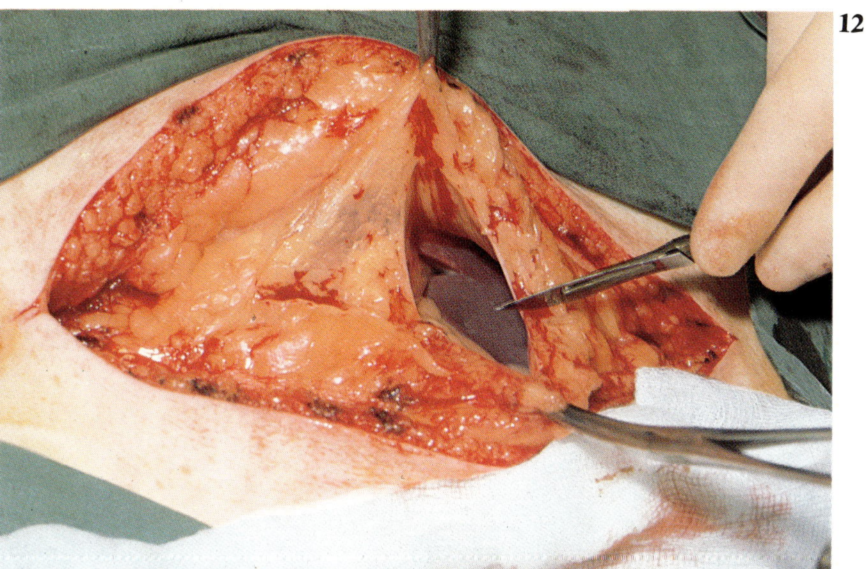

11, 12 and 13 **The peritoneum is incised and opened along the length of the wound.**

13

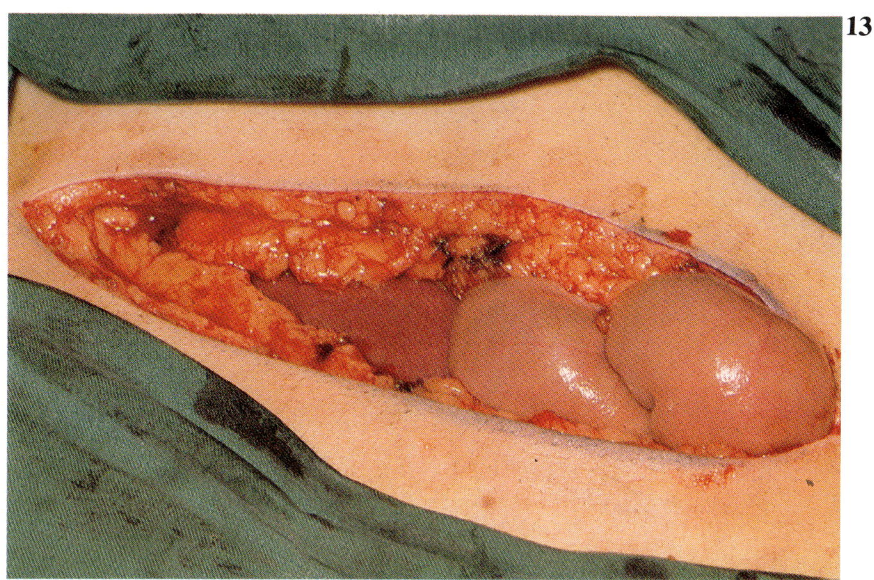

14 The wound is opened and the greater omentum displaced inferiorly.

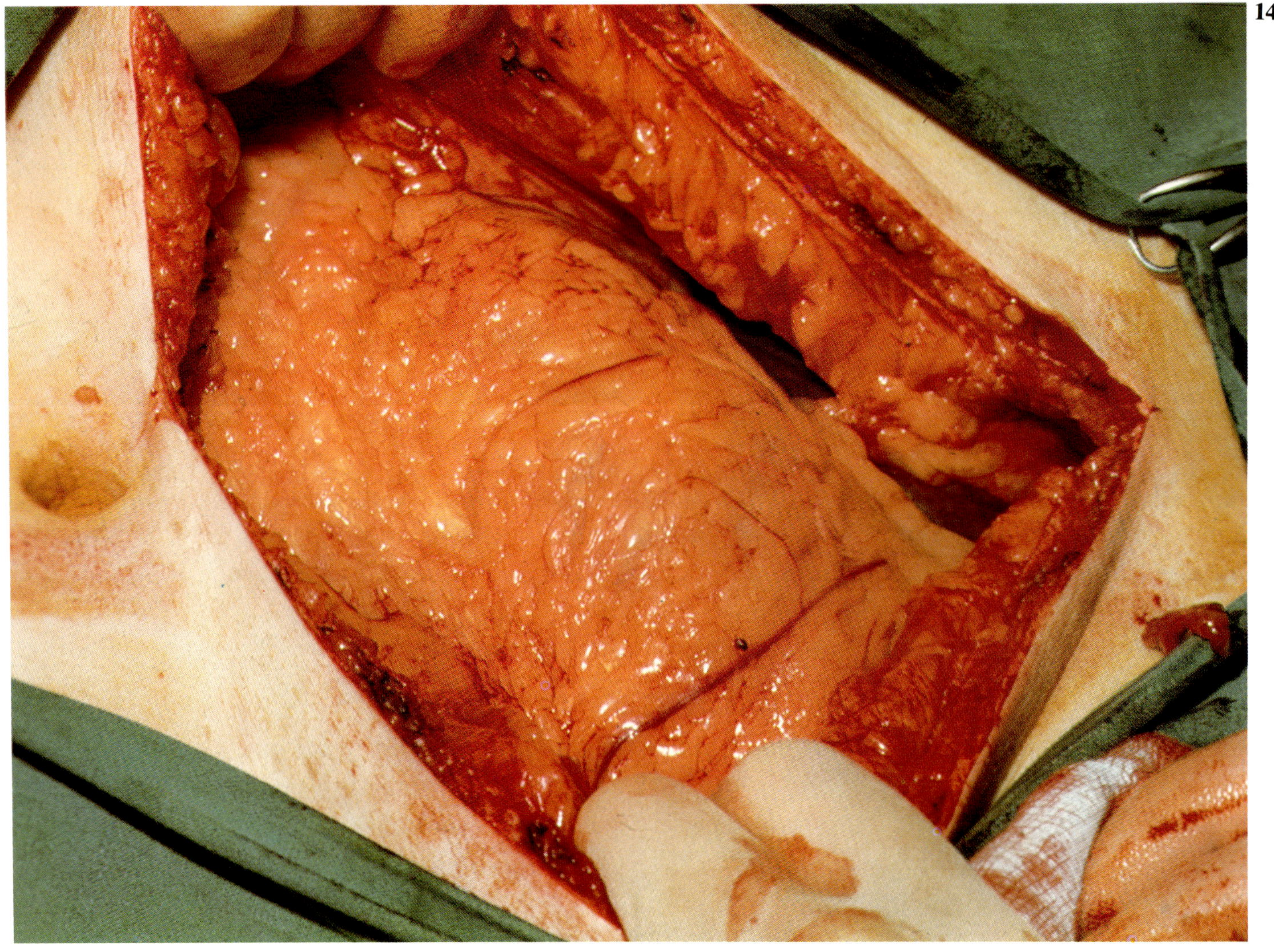
14

Diagnosis of ulceration

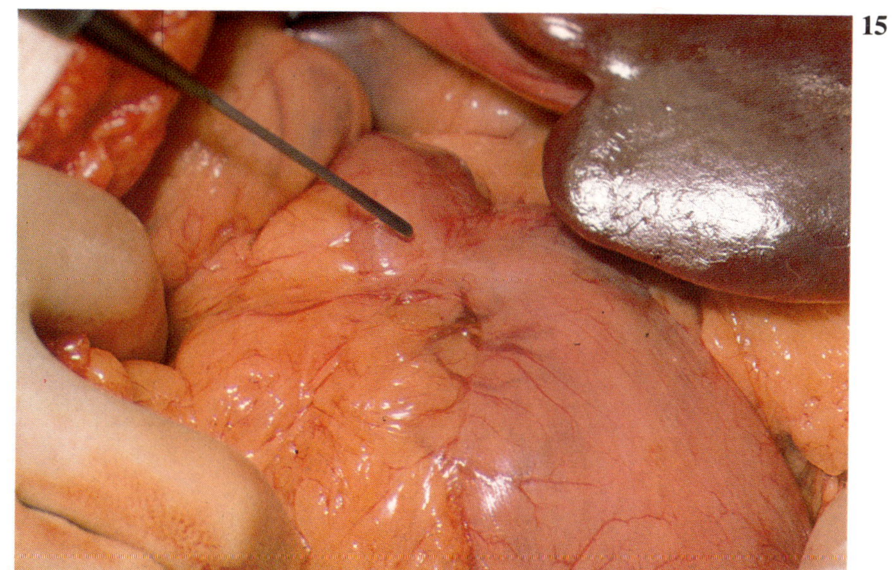

15

15 and 16 **The diagnosis of duodenal ulceration is confirmed by inspection** of the serosal surface of the anterior aspect of the duodenum.

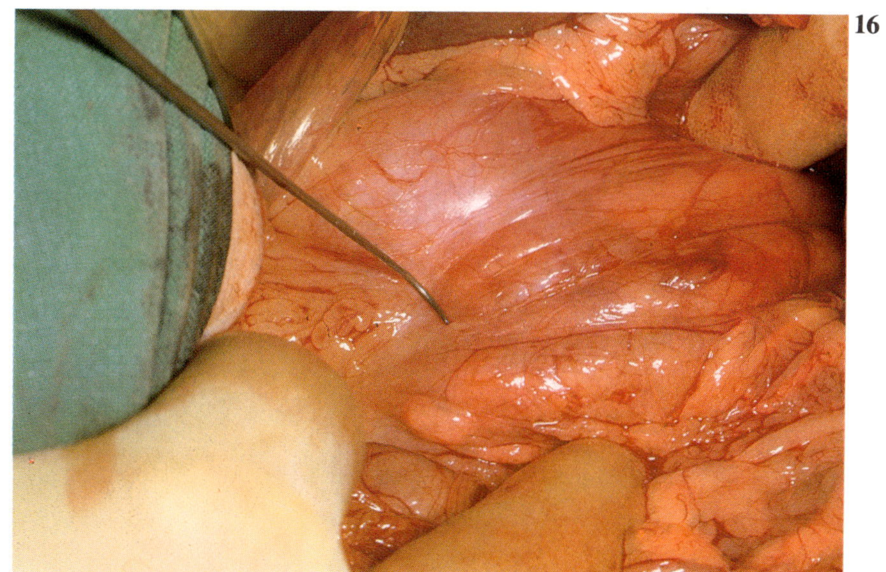

16

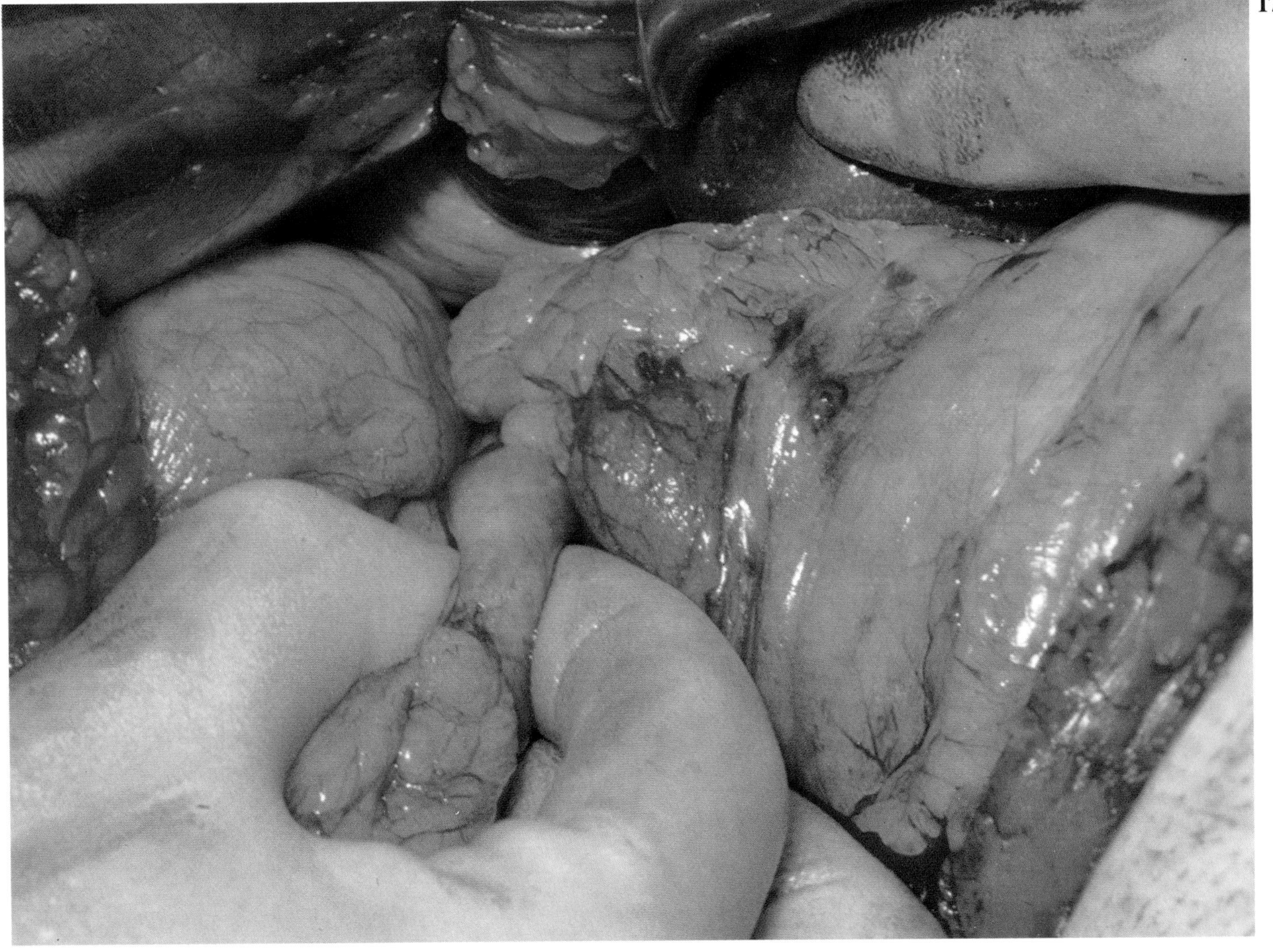

17 The pylorus is palpated for evidence of stenosis, a severe degree of which precludes pylorus-preserving surgery.

18 The gallbladder is palpated to exclude concurrent pathology.

18

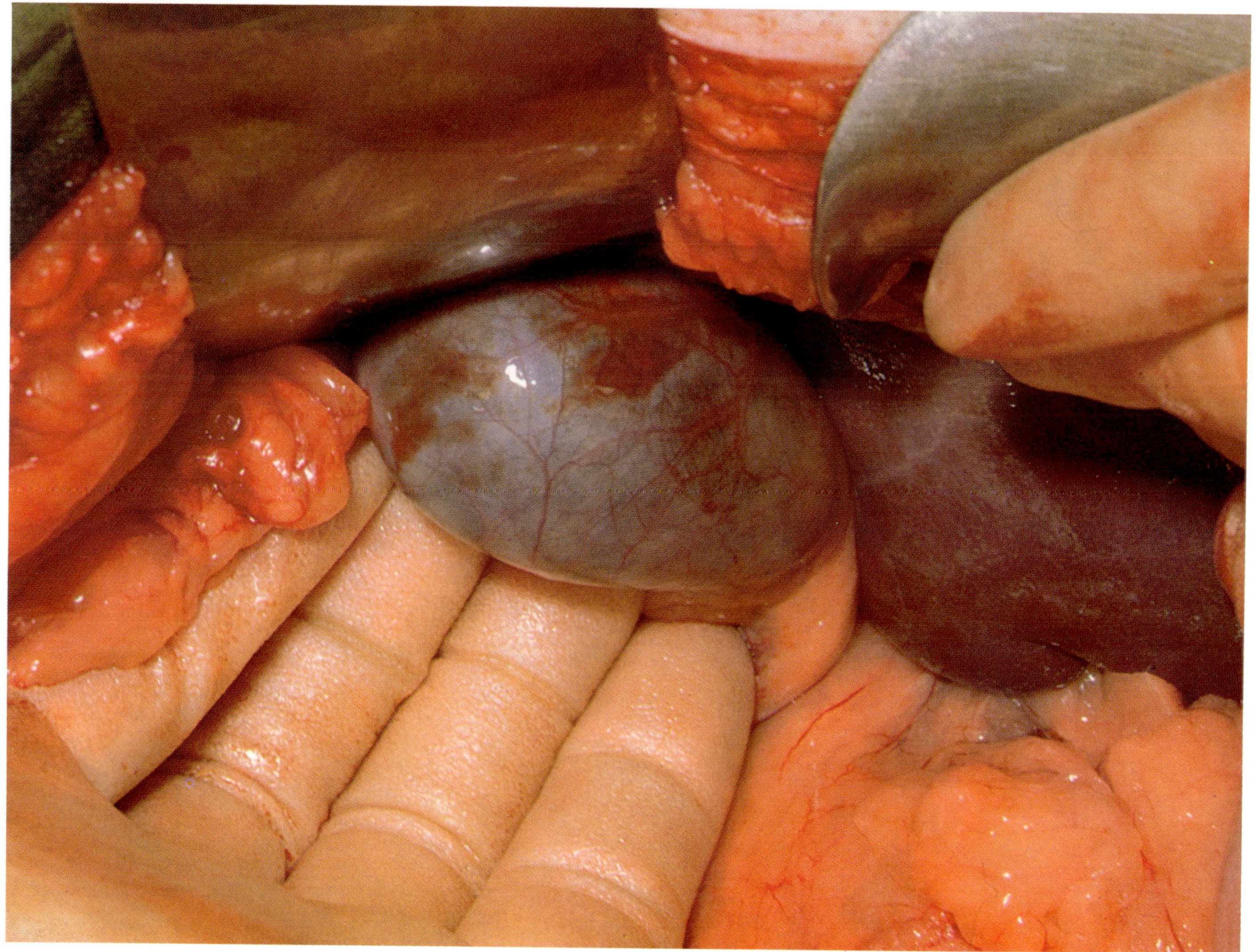

19 The left lobe of the liver is retracted caudally.

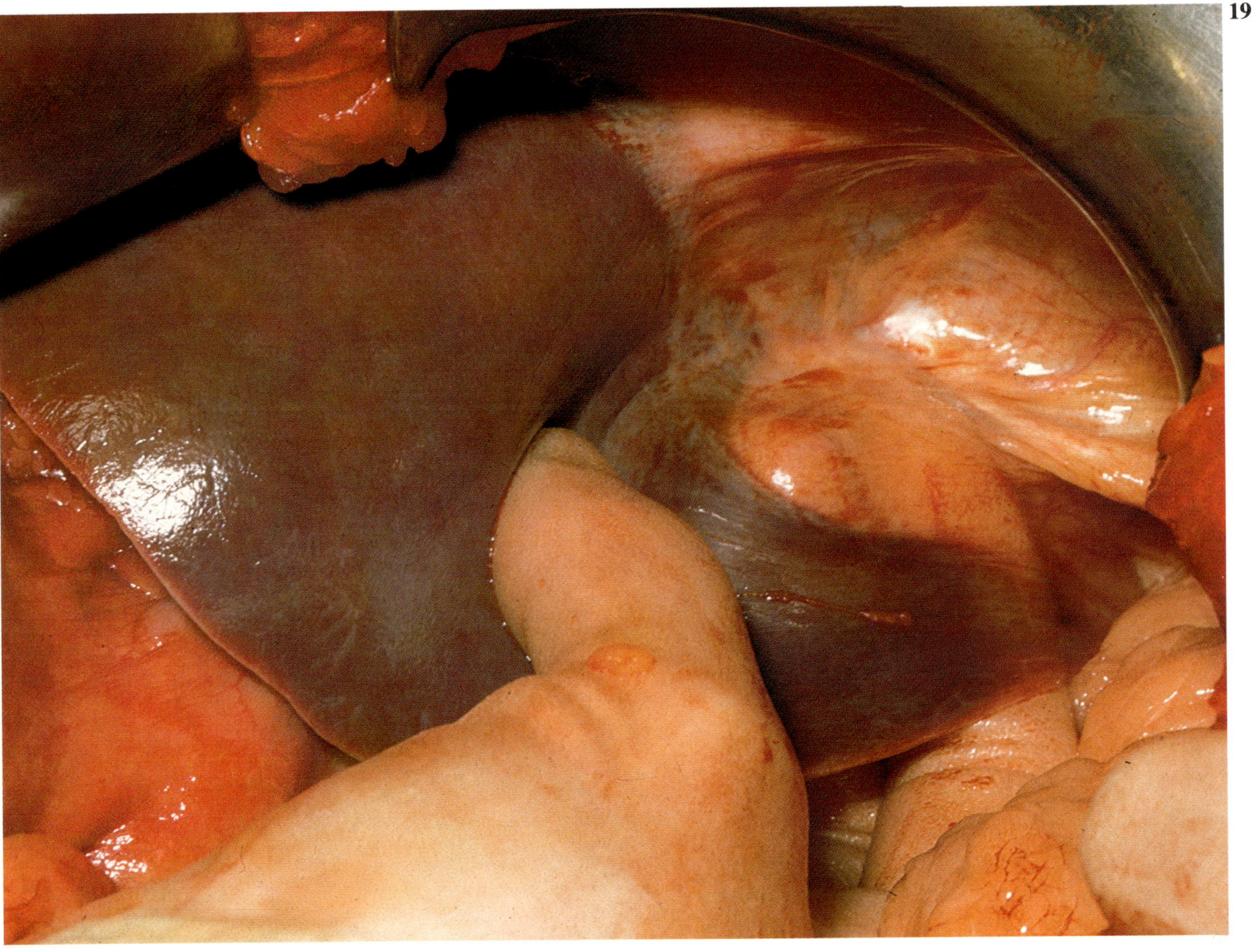

19

20 The left triangular ligament is incised.

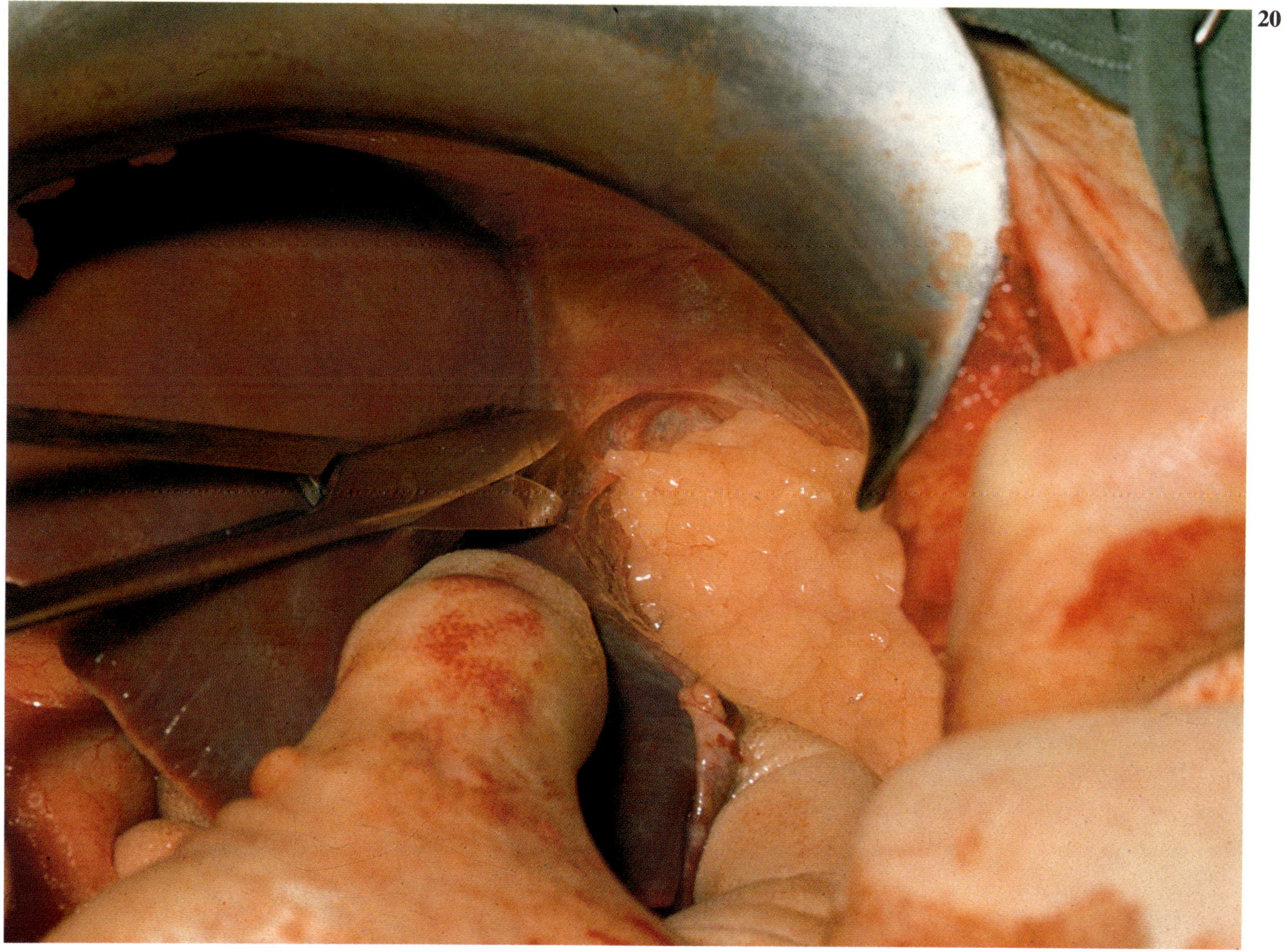
20

21 The left lobe of the liver is retracted to the right to expose the undersurface of the diaphragm and the inferior phrenic vein, at the site of the peritoneal reflection, which extends from the undersurface of the diaphragm onto the posterior abdominal wall.

21

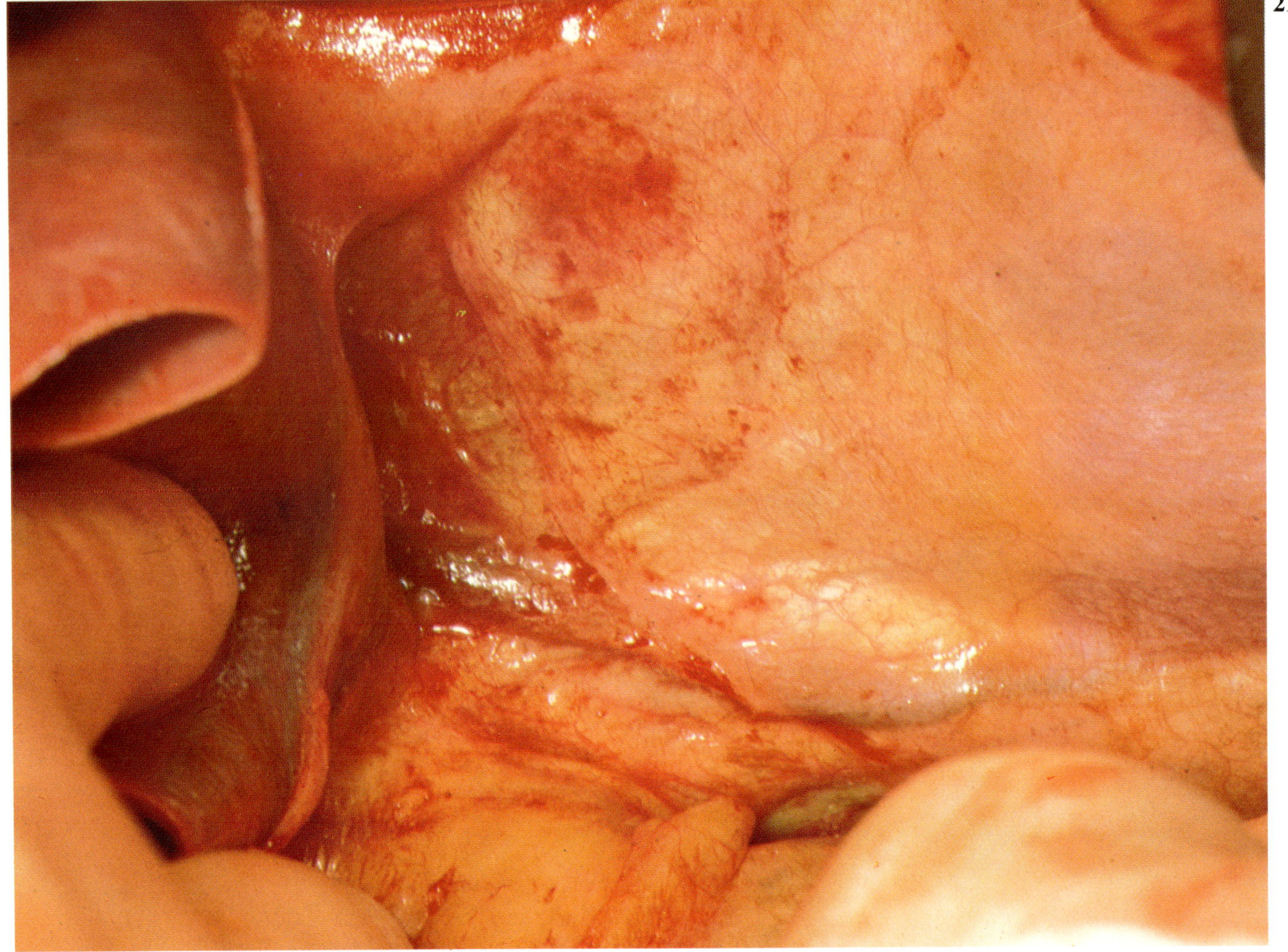

22 The peritoneum overlying the anterior aspect of the oesophagus is incised with scissors, care being taken not to cut the inferior phrenic vein which can be displaced.

22

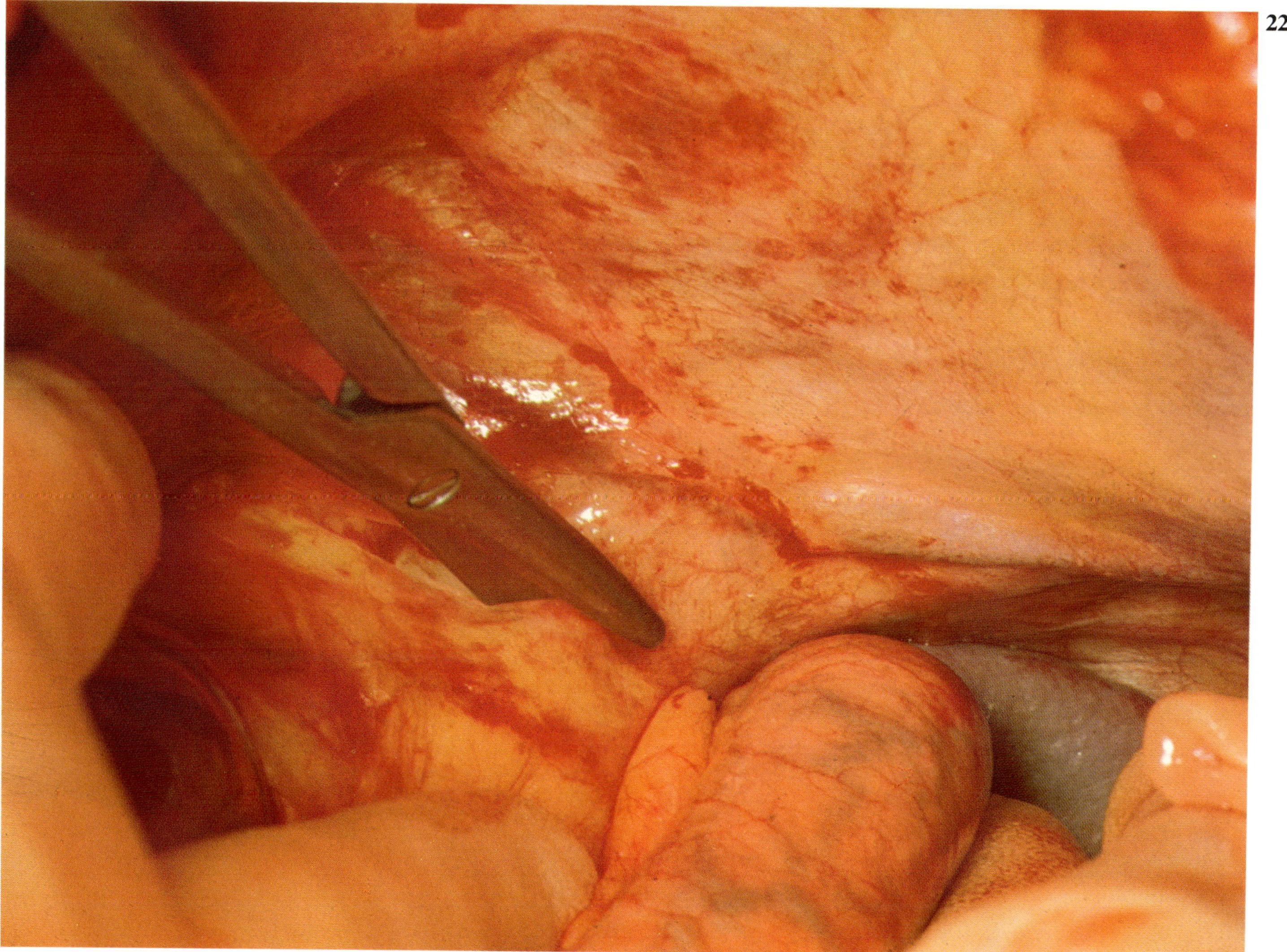

23 **The peritoneum is reflected to expose the anterior aspect of the oesophagus which is lifted forwards.**

23

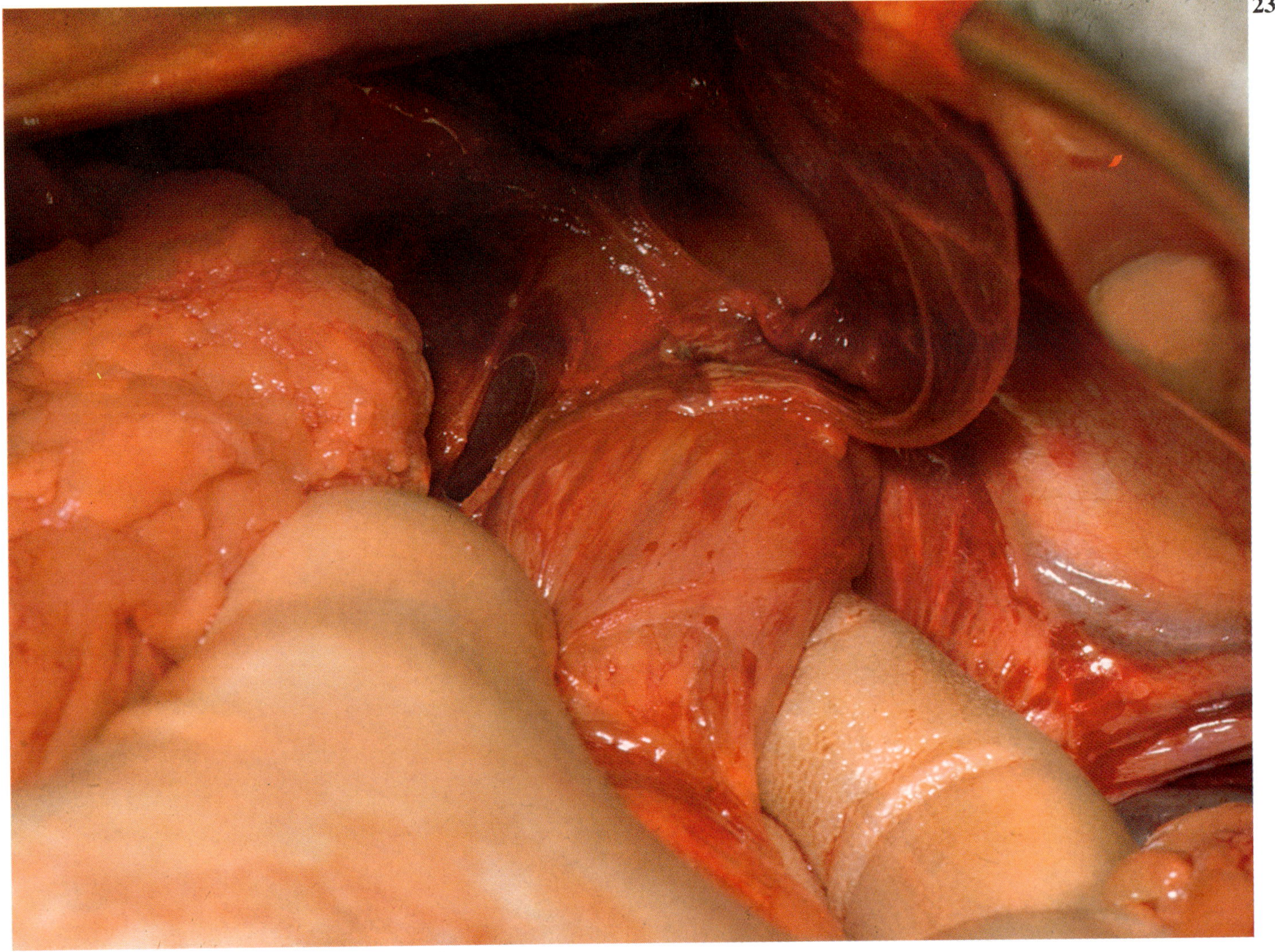

24 The index finger of the right hand is insinuated around the oesophagus.

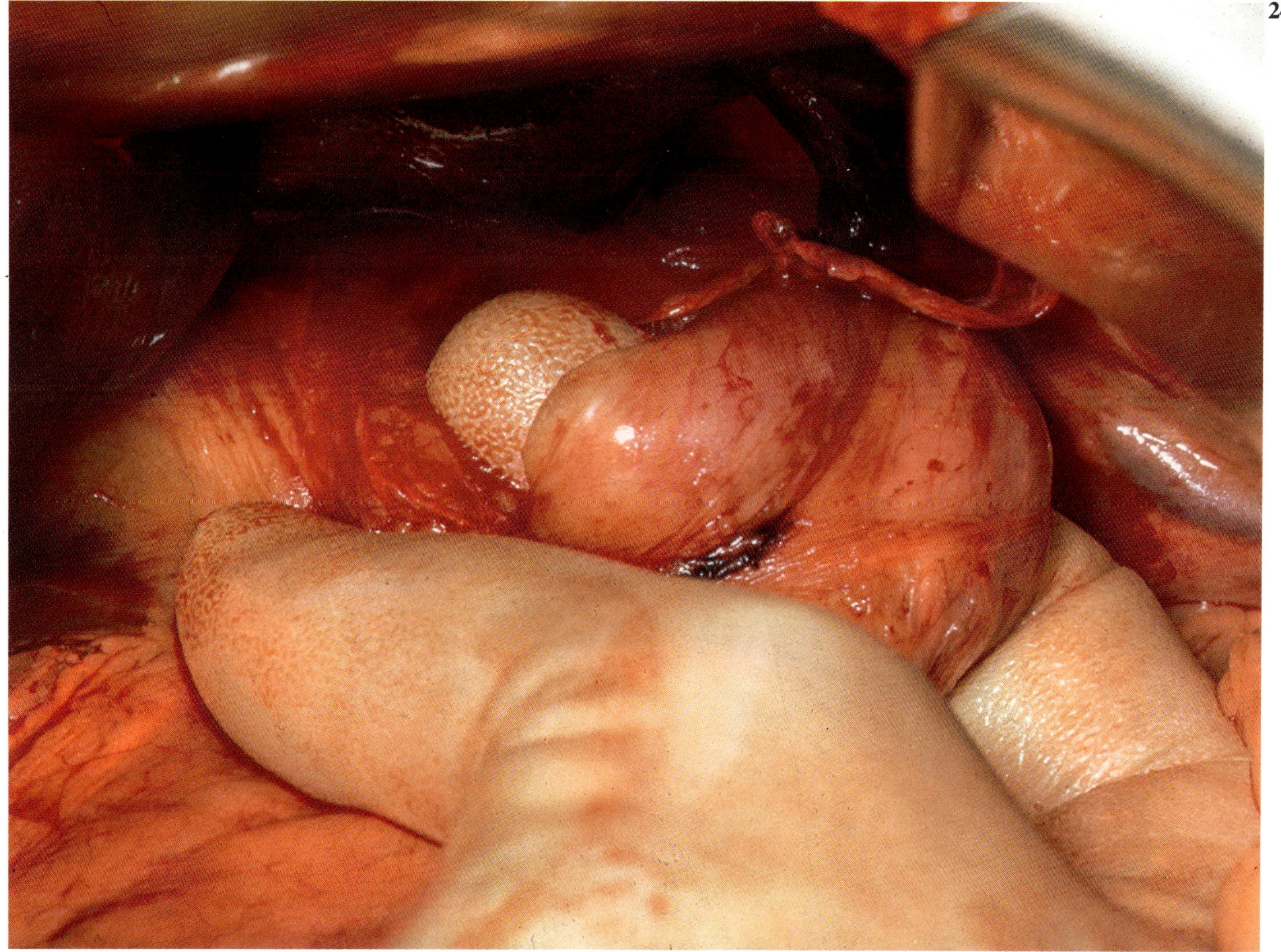

24

25 The lower oesophagus is further mobilised by placing the index and middle fingers behind it and gently spreading the areolar tissue.

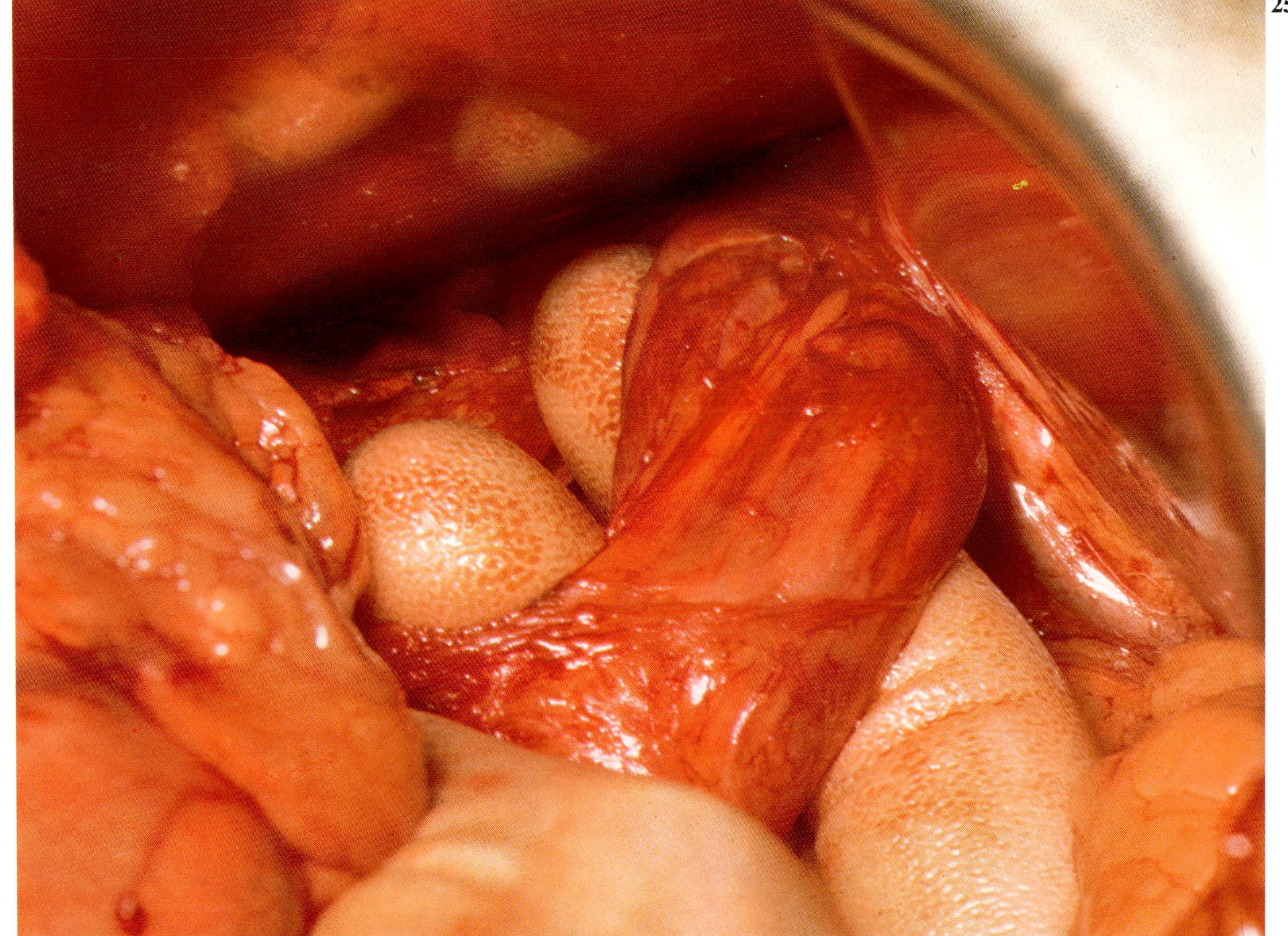

25

Anterior vagus dissected

26 The anterior vagus, which is adherent to the anterior wall of the oesophagus, is dissected free from this structure. A flimsy film of areolar tissue binding the nerve to the oesophagus is seen stretched over the tip of the index finger.

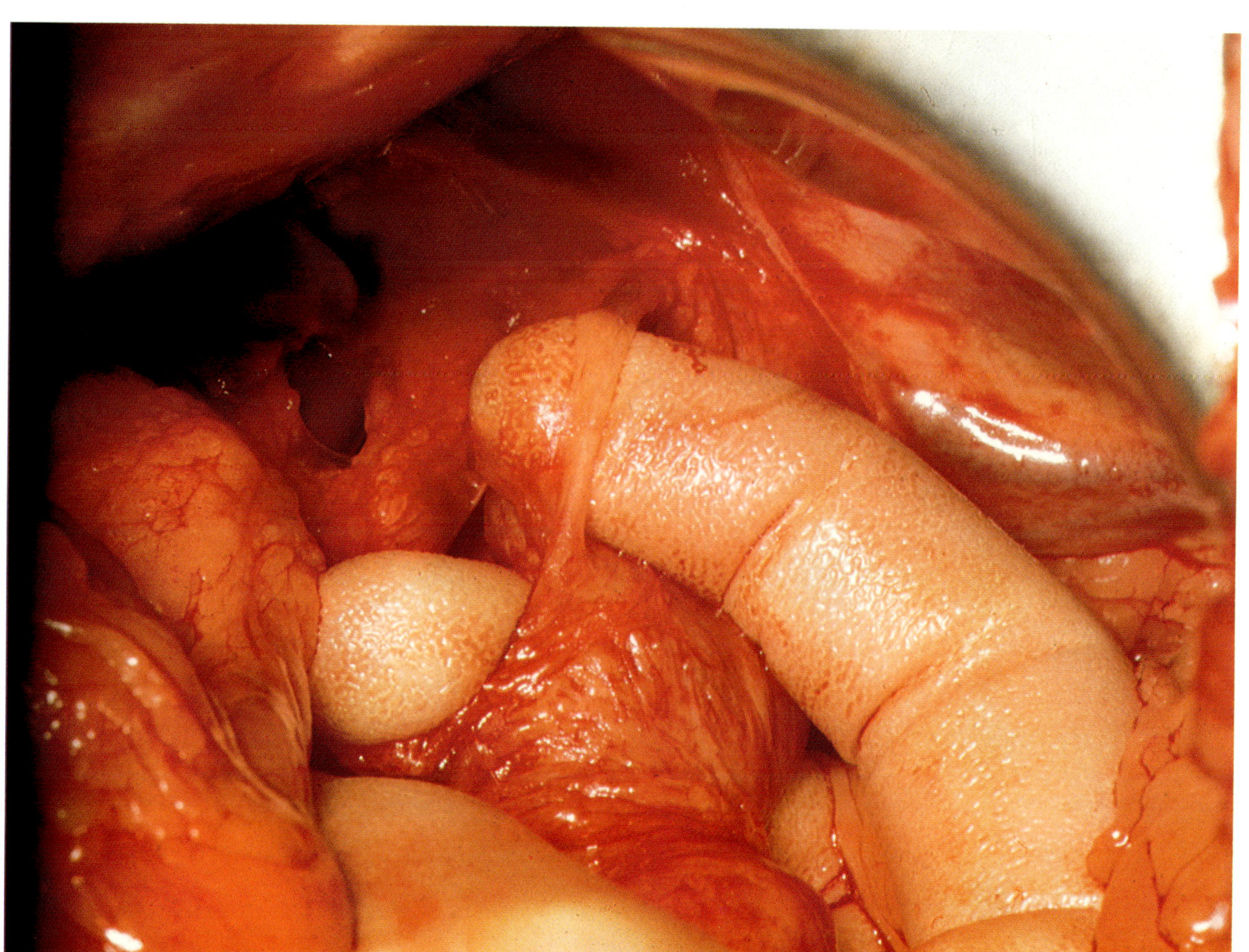

26

27

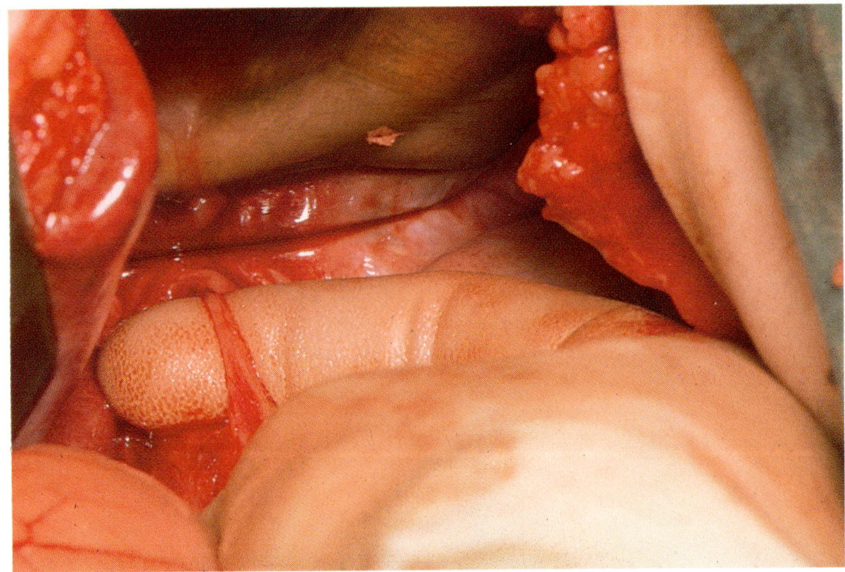

28

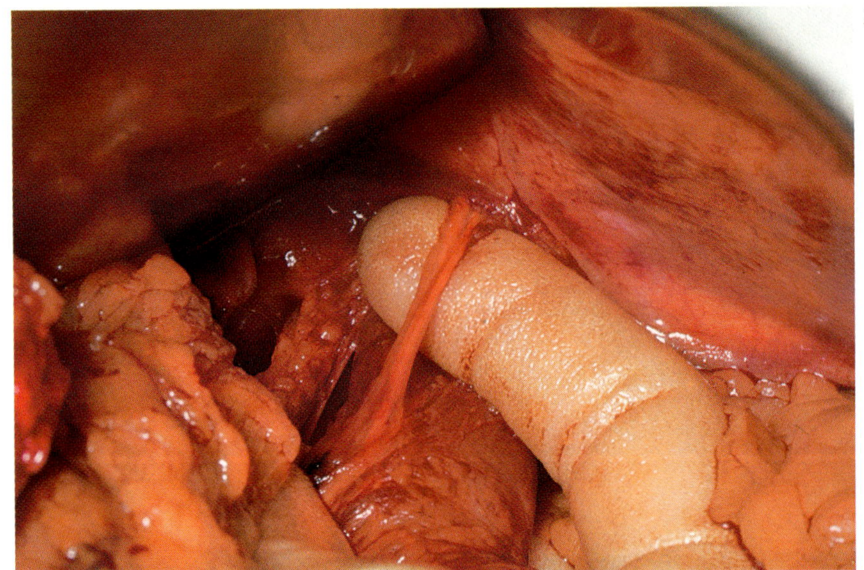

27 The anterior vagus is further mobilised by blunt dissection.

28 The nerve should be mobilised up to the level of the diaphragm.

29 Any sheaths of areolar tissue between the nerve and the oesophagus are incised with scissors, as these contain nerve fibres running from the anterior vagal trunk into the oesophageal wall and possibly down, through this structure, to the parietal cell area of the stomach. The main anterior nerve can always be definitely identified by its spatulate lower end, shown here stretched over the index finger.

29

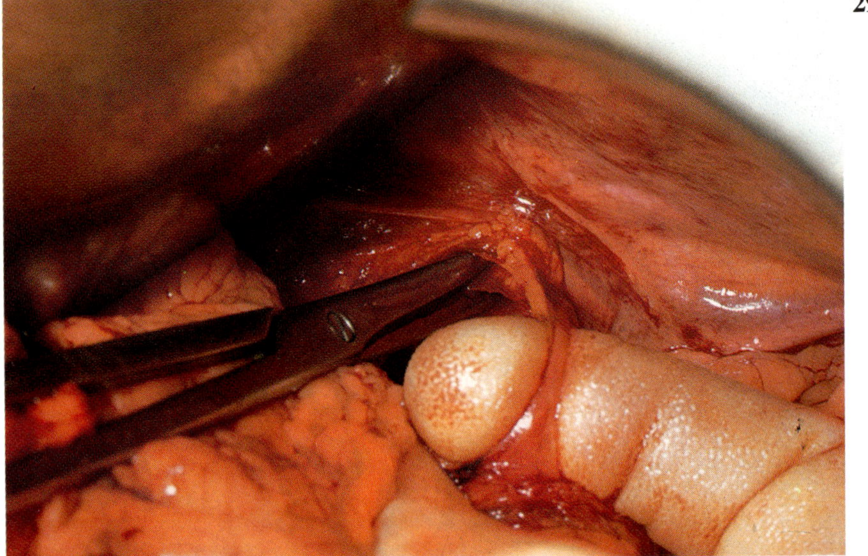

30

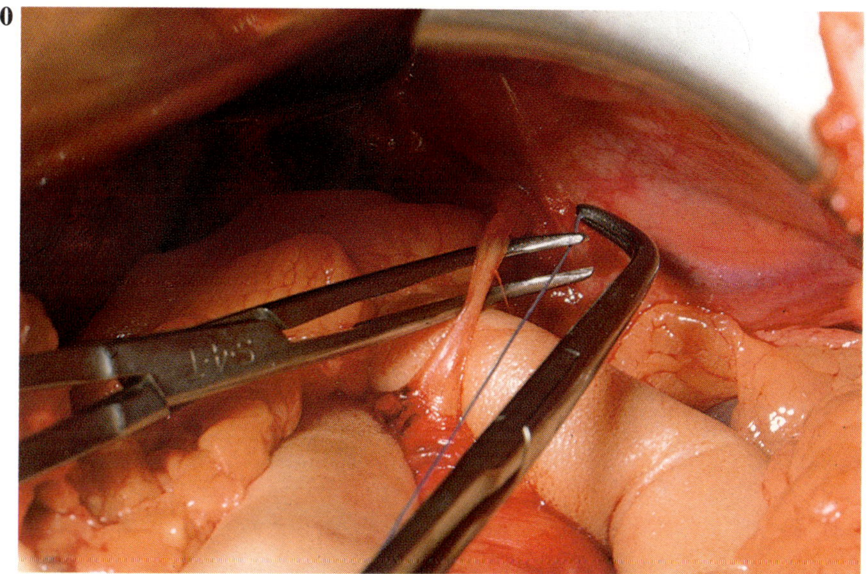

31

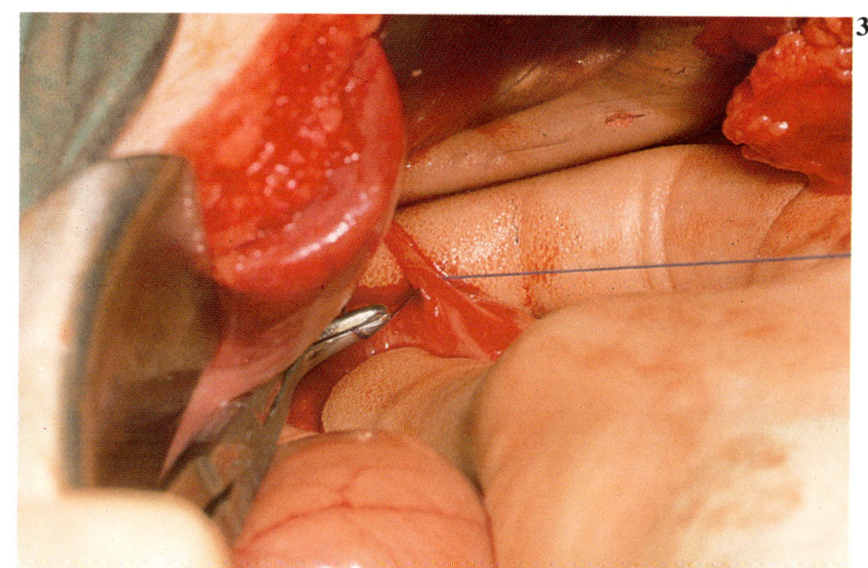

30, 31 and 32 A suture to be used as a sling, is next placed around the fully mobilised anterior vagus nerve.

32

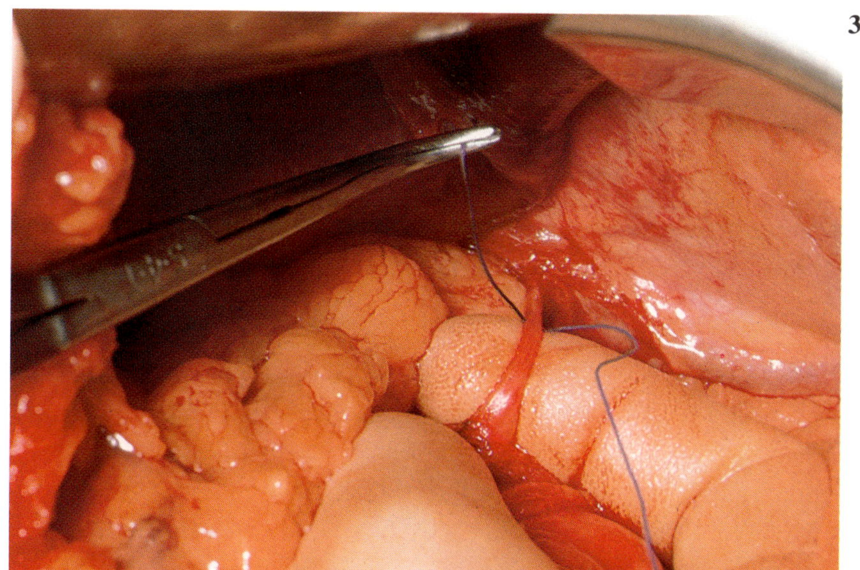

33

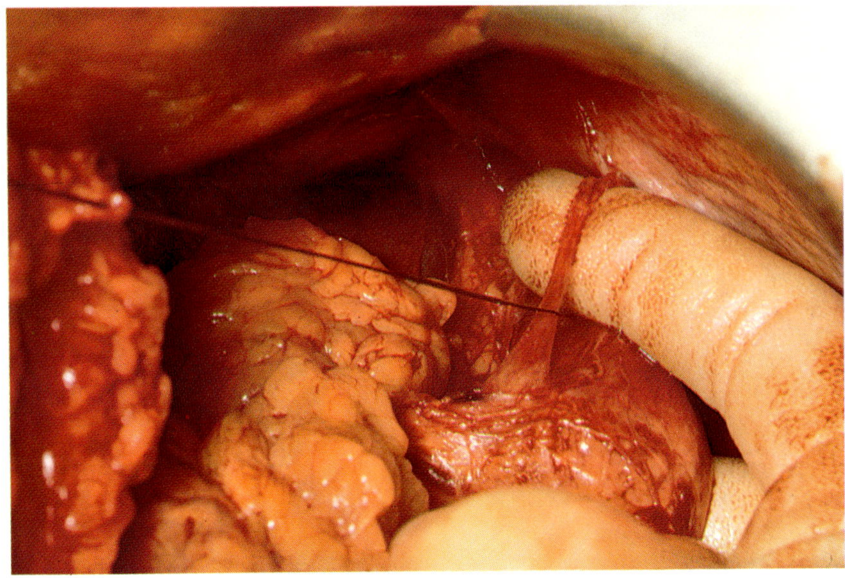

34

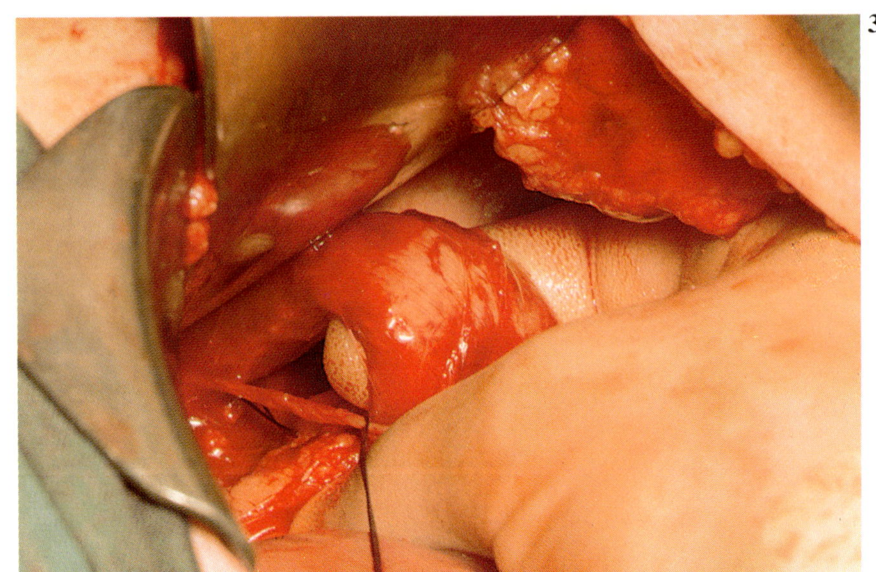

33 and 34 By applying gentle traction to this sling the anterior vagus nerve can be retracted clear of the oesophagus.

Preservation of the anterior vagal trunk is of fundamental importance in this procedure.

35

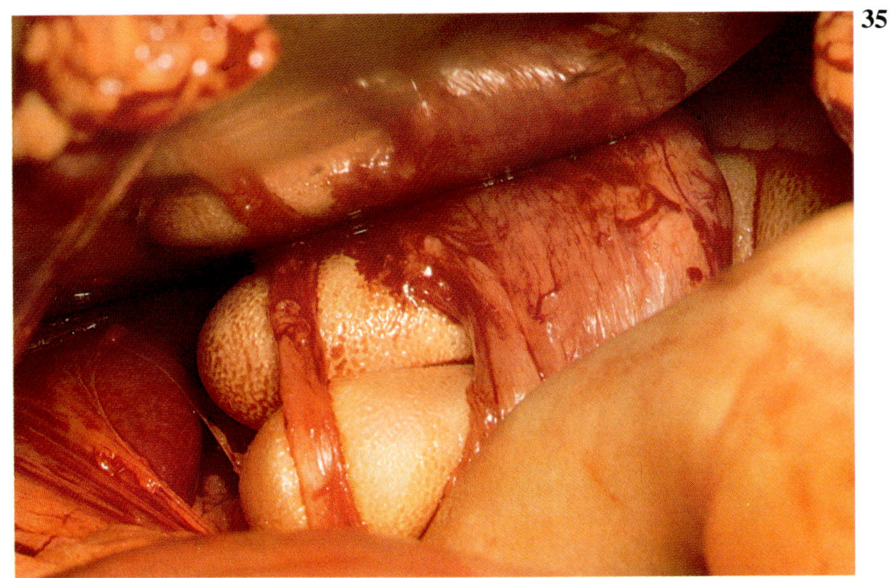

35 The posterior vagus nerve trunk, which lies posteromedial to and separate from the oesophagus, is next identified by sweeping the index finger in an arc between the aorta and the right crus of the diaphragm.

Posterior nerve mobilised, diathermised and cut

36

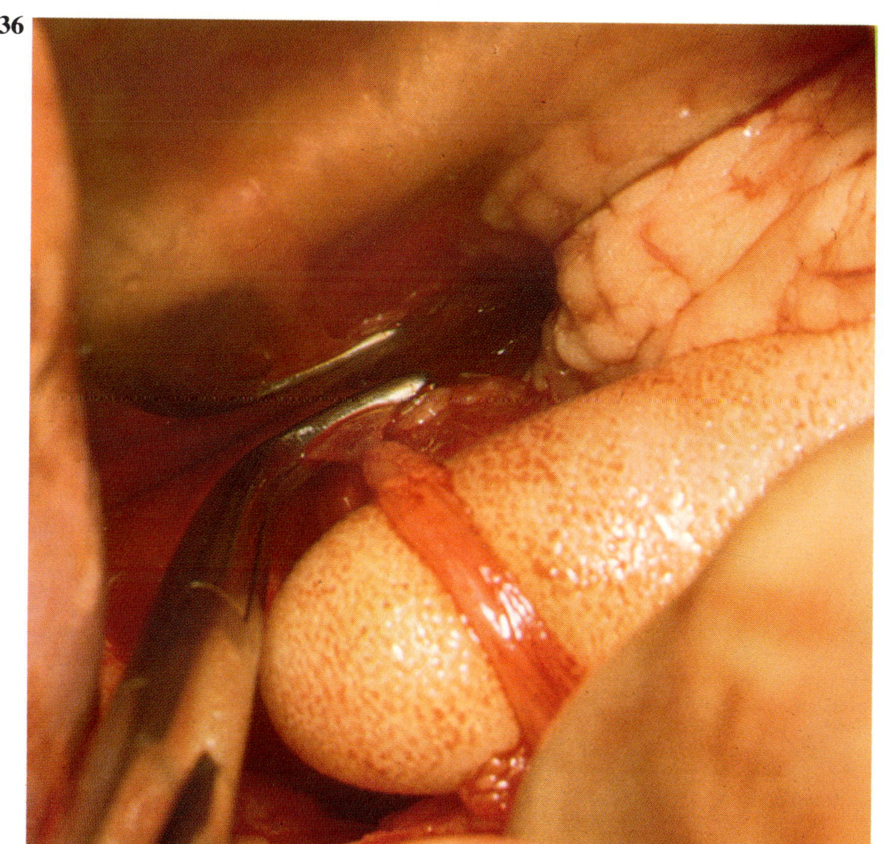

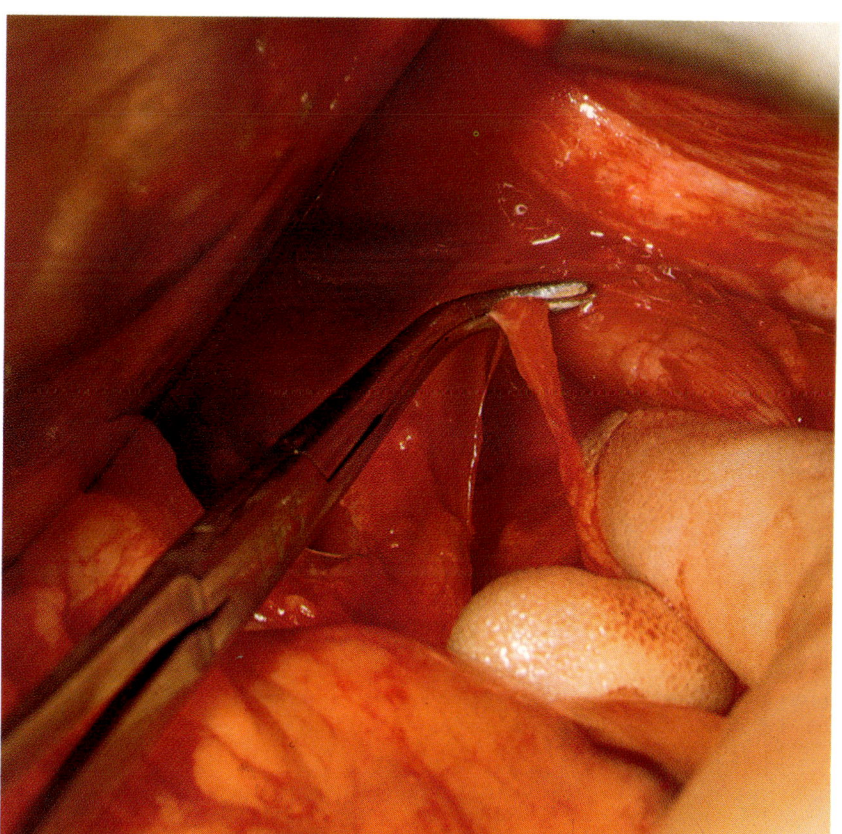

37

36 and 37 The posterior nerve is mobilised up to the level of the oesophageal hiatus and clamped at this level with a pair of Lahey forceps.

38

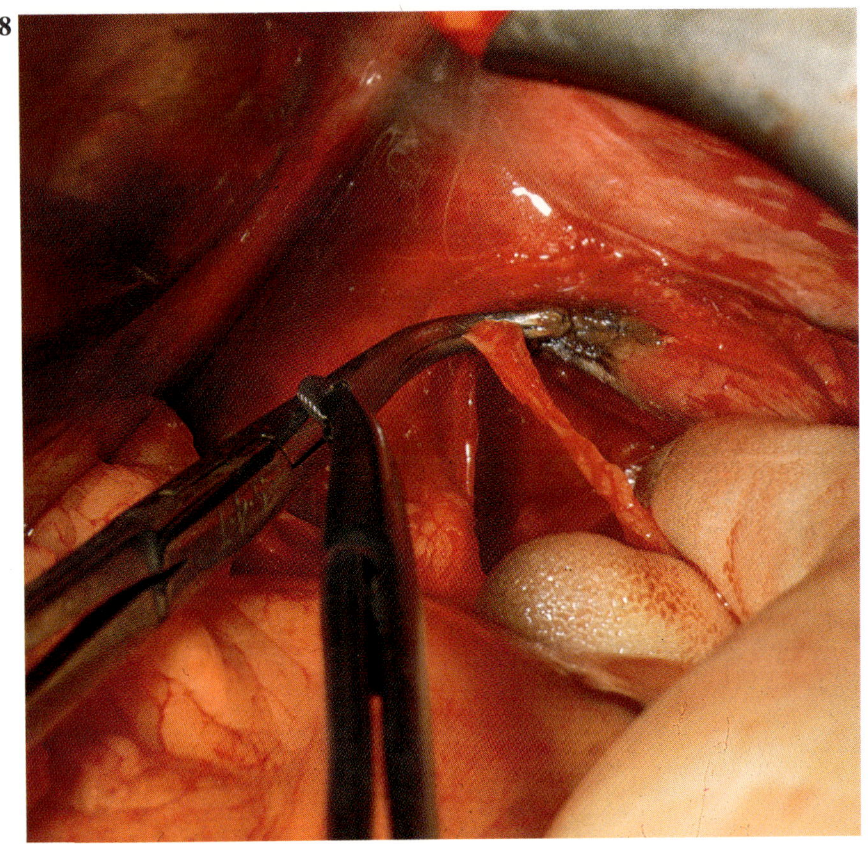

39

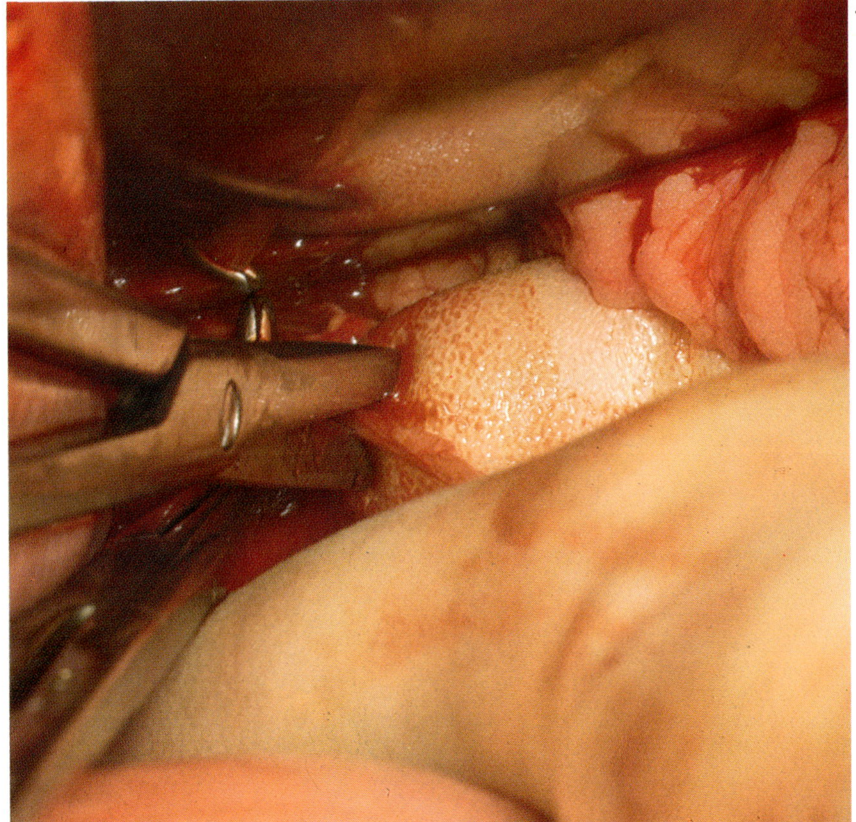

38 and 39 **The nerve is then diathermised and cut.**

40

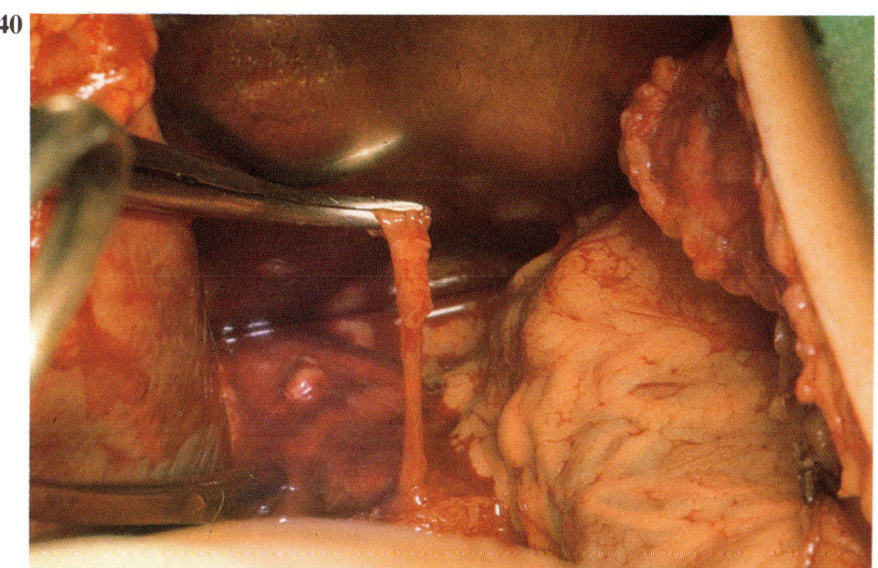

41

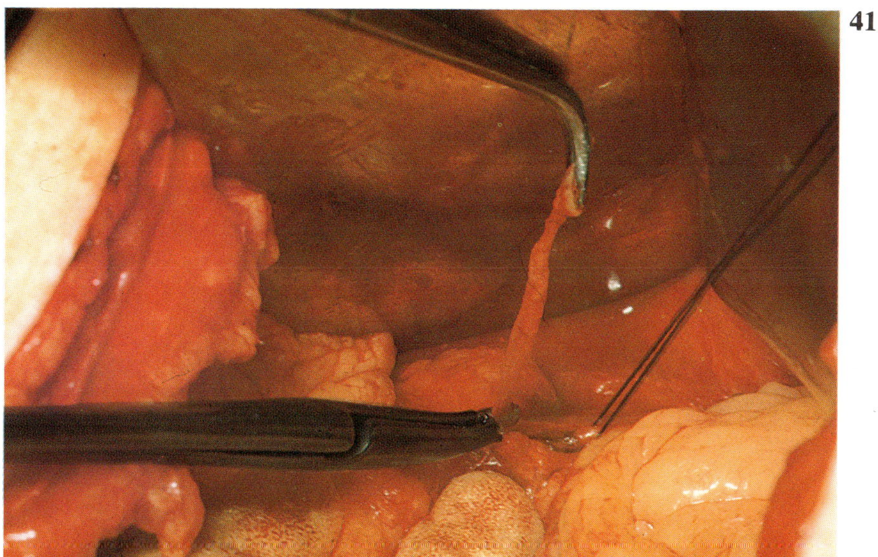

40, 41 and 42 A length of at least two inches of nerve is lifted forwards and again diathermised, and divided well clear of the anterior nerve held in the sling.

42

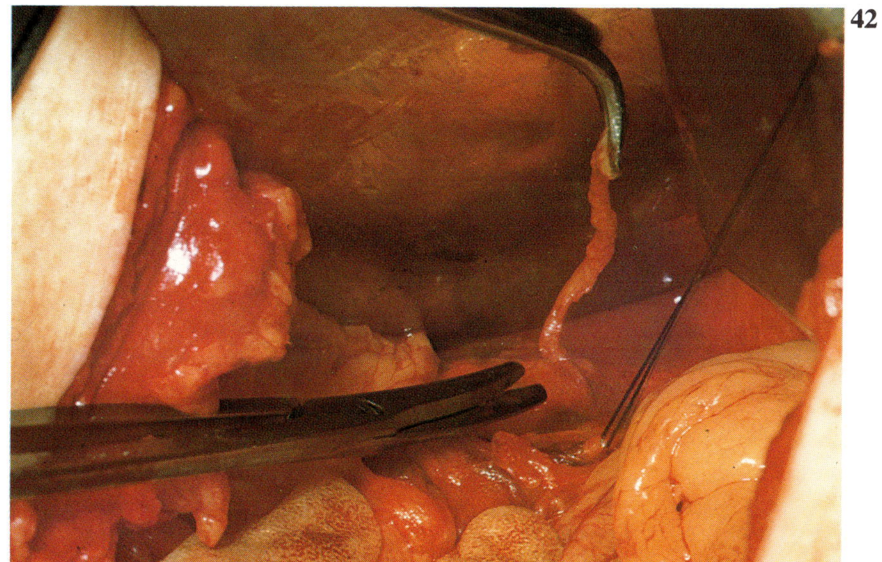

43

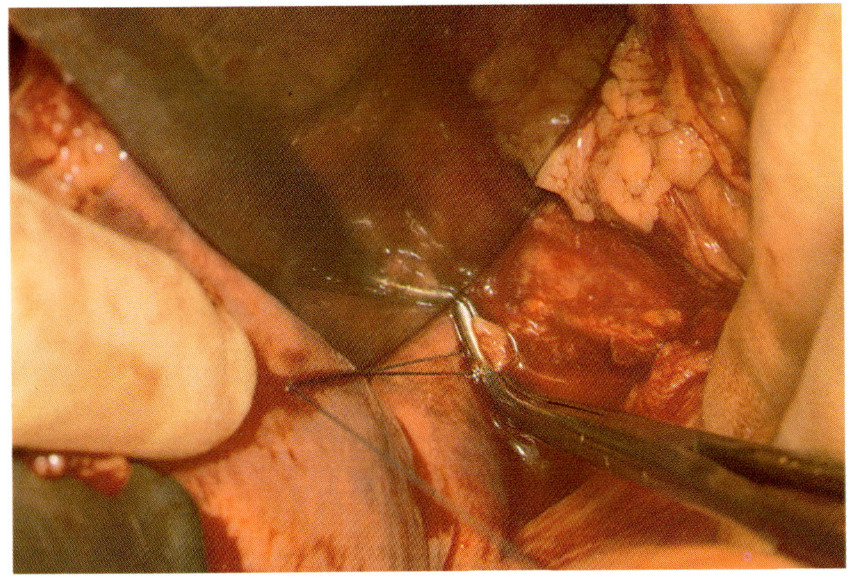

44

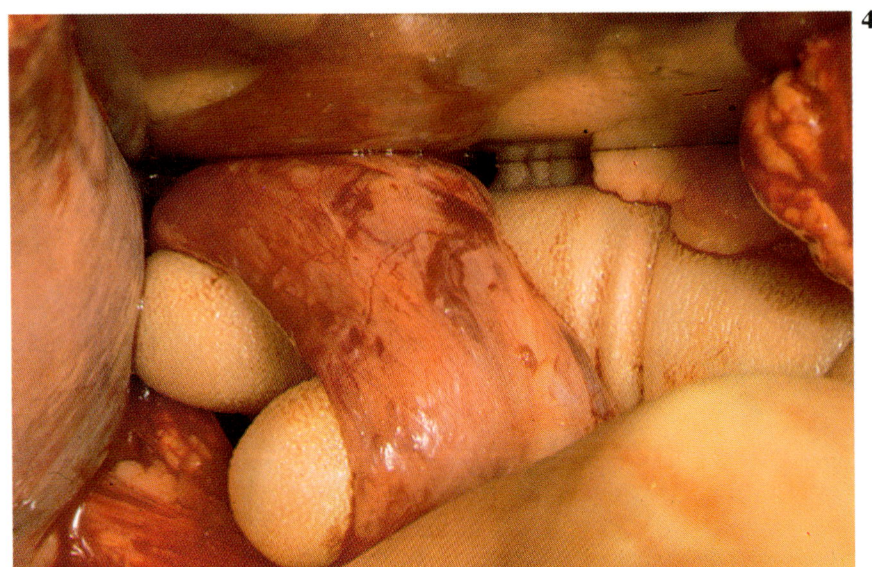

43 The nerve may be ligated rather than diathermised.

44 The lower end of the oesophagus is now exposed along a distance of 5 cm to 6 cm.

45 Several small vagal strands which require division can be seen here.

45

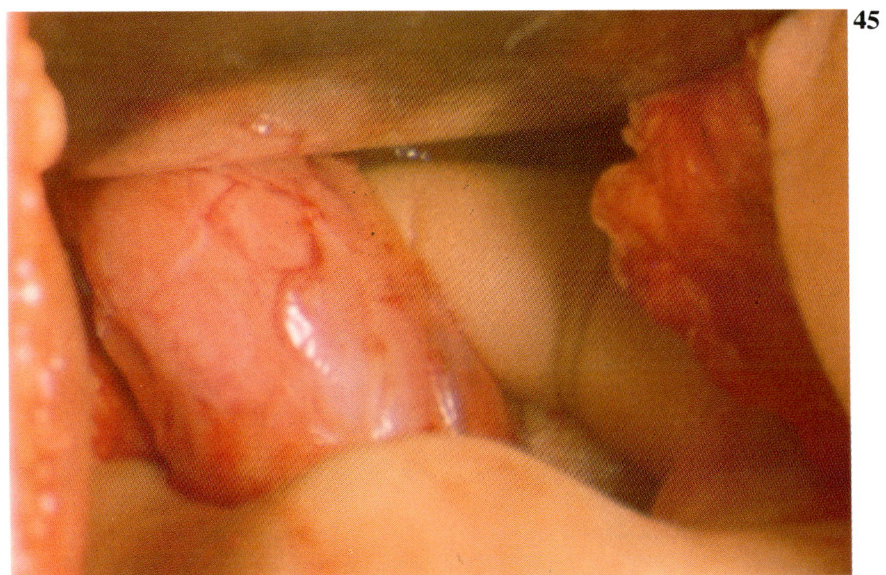

46

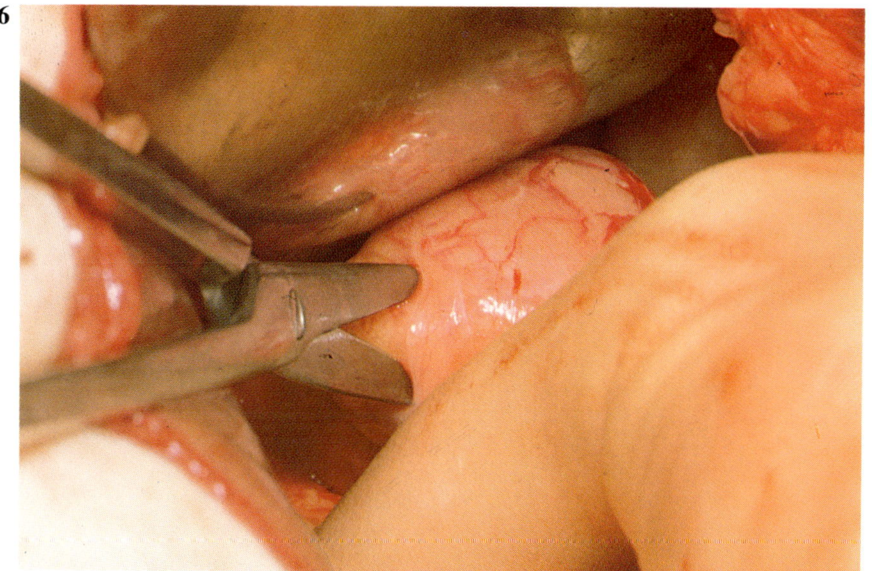

47

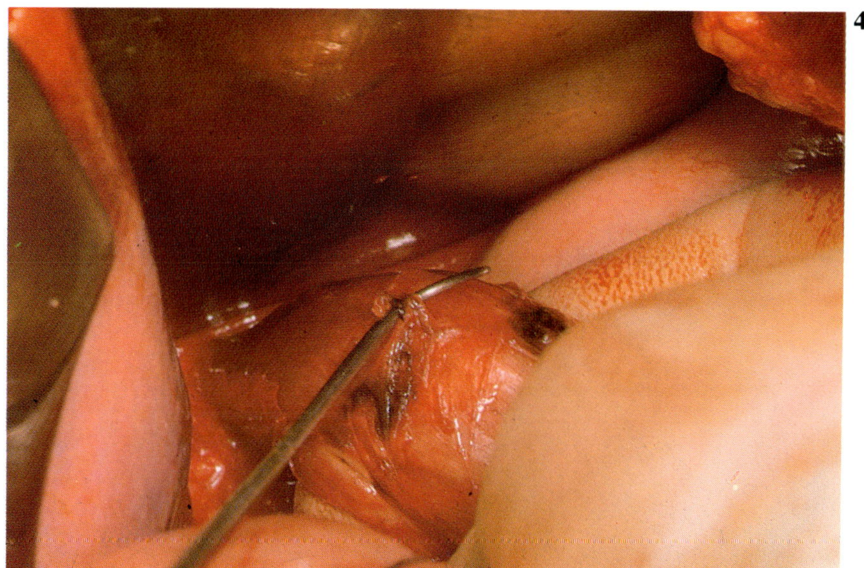

46 These small residual vagal strands running along the lower oesophagus are divided.

47 and 48 Small strands can be picked up with the vagus nerve hook diathermised and divided.

48

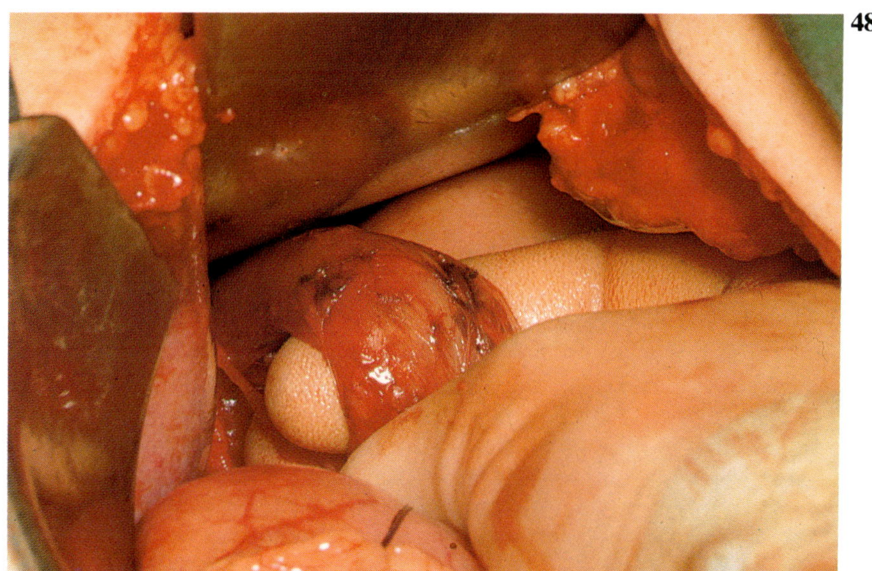

49

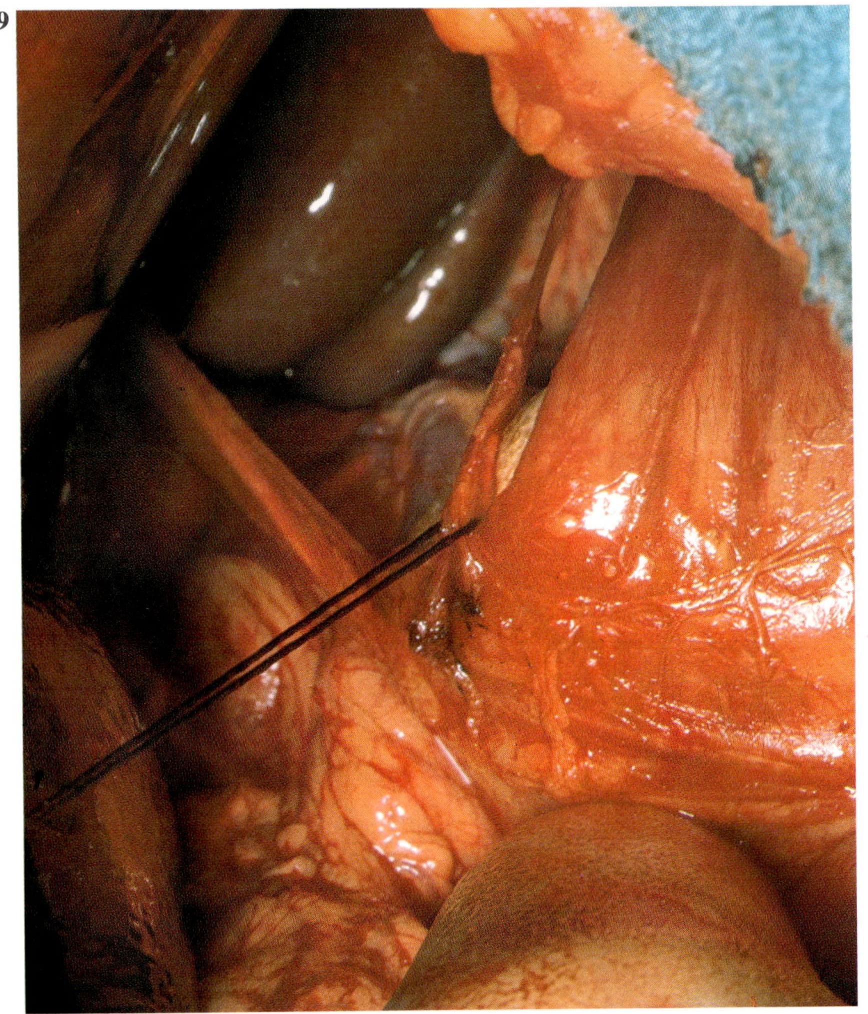

50

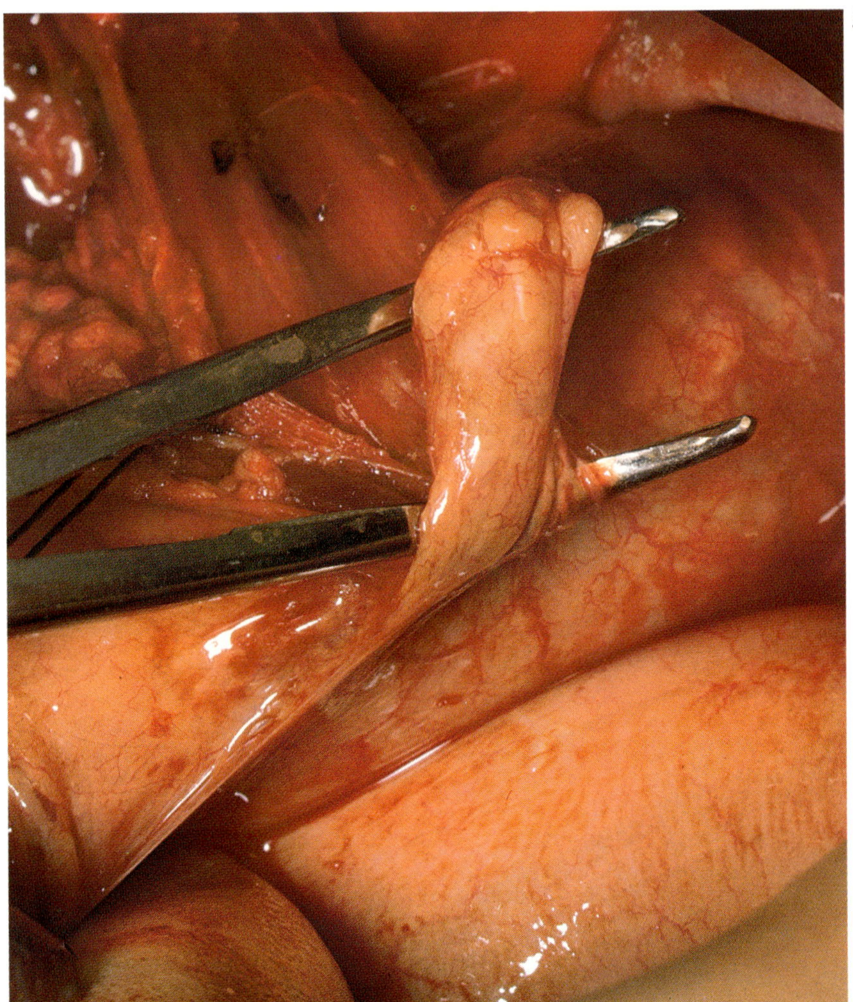

49 Here is the lower oesophagus cleared of residual vagal fibres with the anterior vagal trunk to the left and the hepatic branches of the anterior vagus running horizontally to the left. In the lower area of the field beneath the surgeon's index finger runs a constantly placed, transversely disposed, fibro-fatty, neurovascular bundle.

50 This bundle requires division as it contains branches from the anterior vagus. It is here being mobilised by a pair of Lahey forceps.

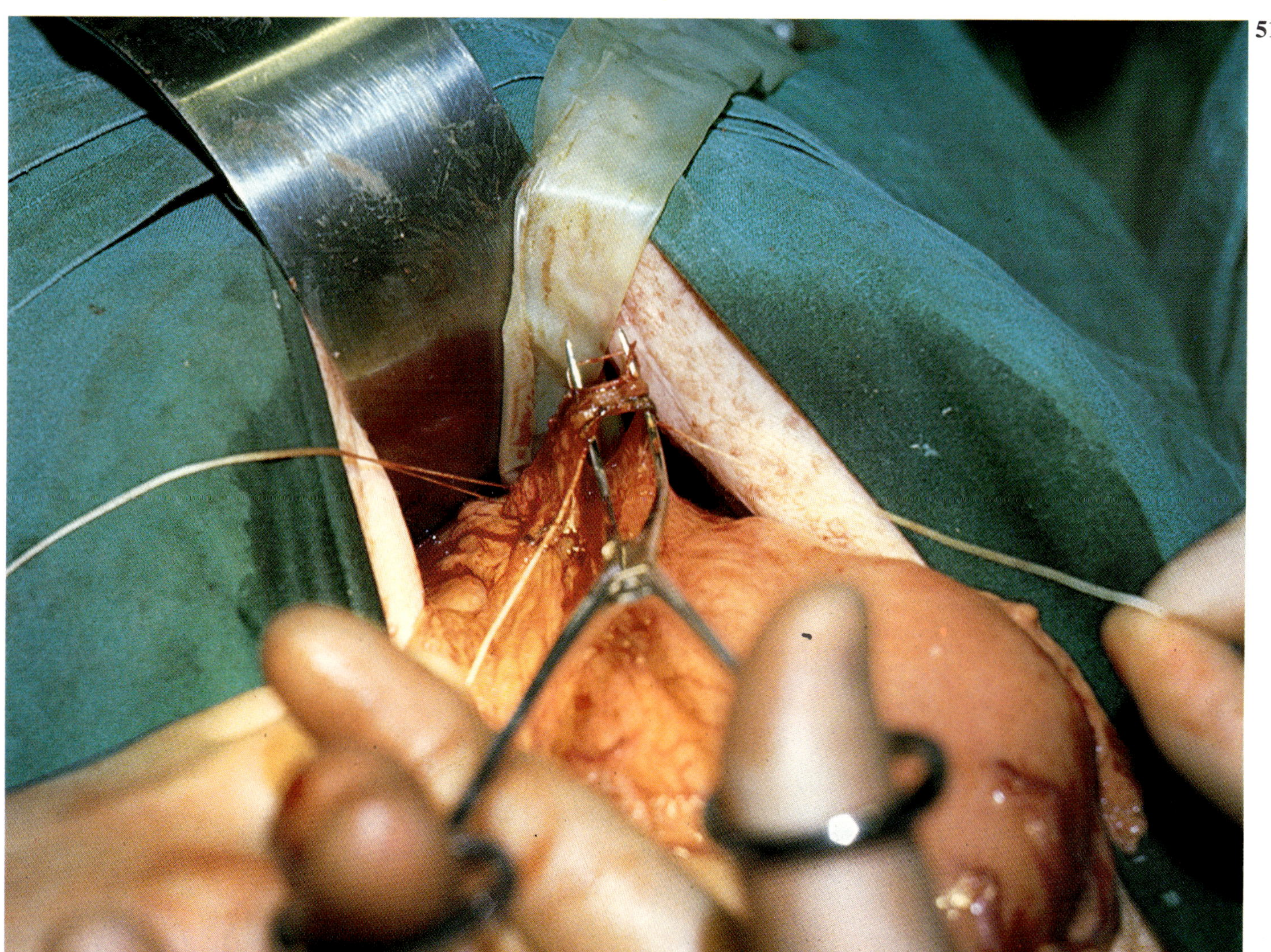
51

51 Mobilisation of this bundle may be facilitated by the use of a pair of double aneurysm forceps, as shown here.

52

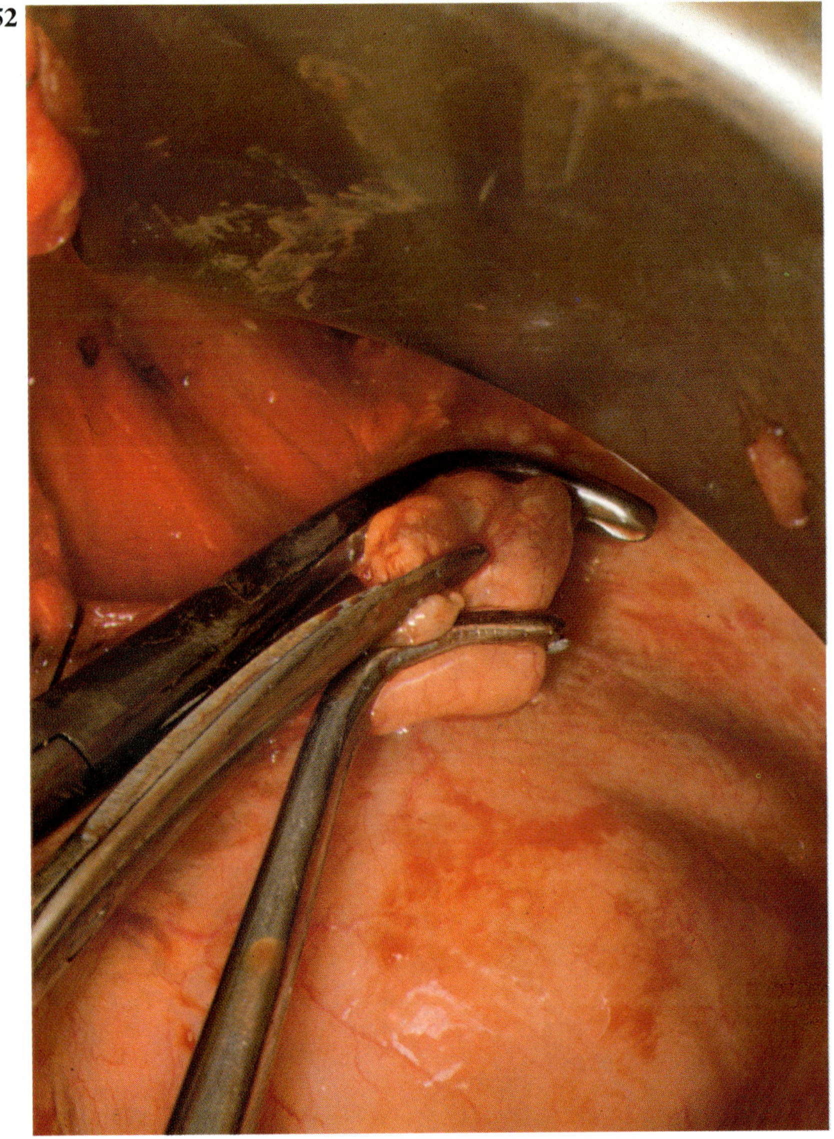

53

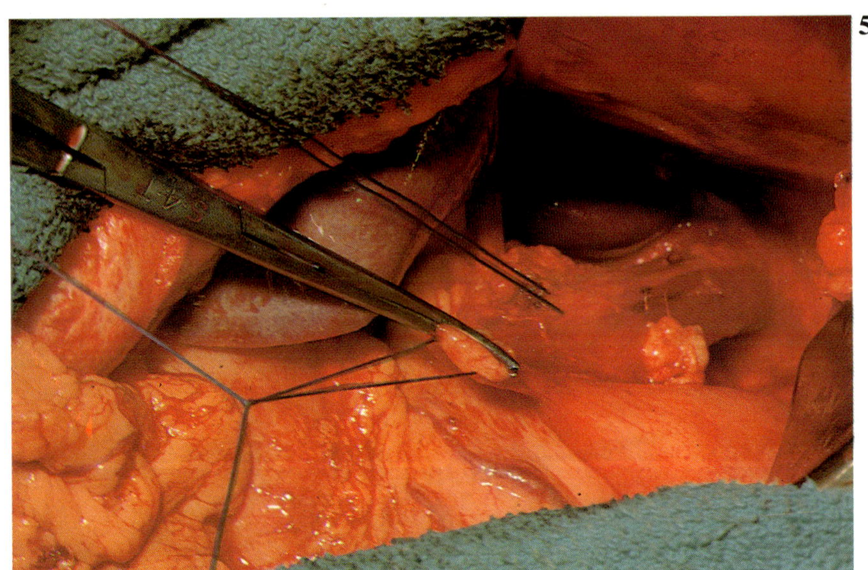

54

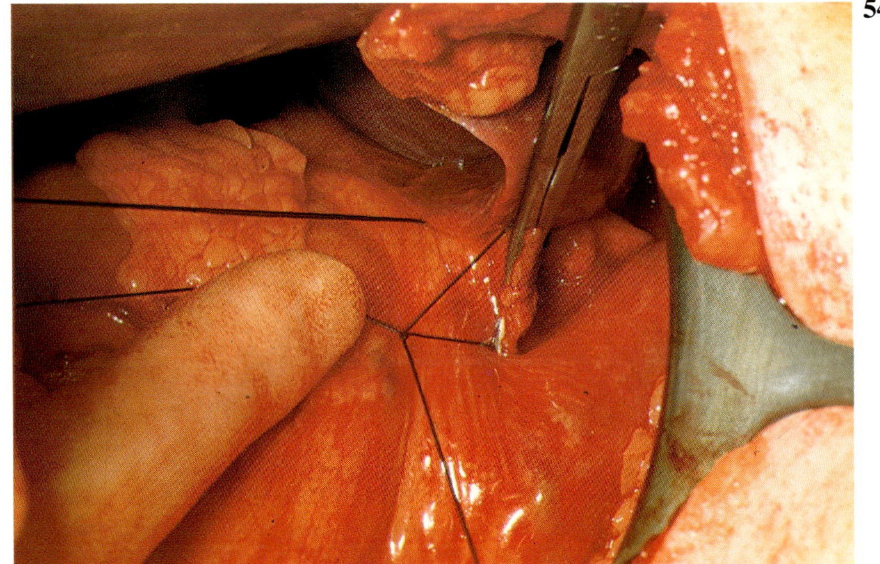

52, 53 and 54 **This bundle is divided and ligated.**

Serosal surface of stomach exposed

55 The serosal surface of the proximal end of the stomach is now exposed.

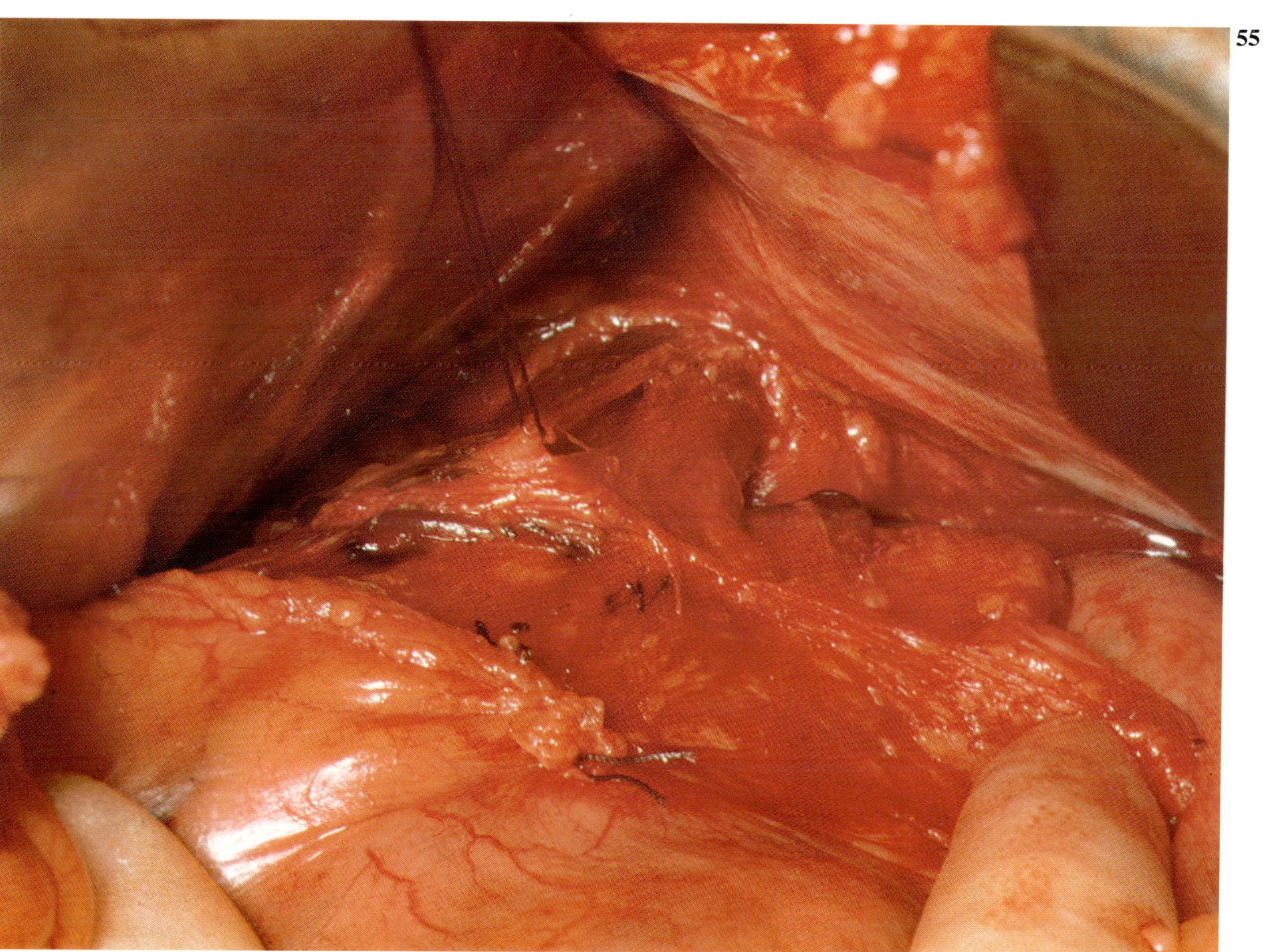

55

56 Regarding the seromyotomy three anatomical factors are worthy of consideration:

1 There is no particular predilection for branches of the nerve of Latarjet to accompany vessels along the walls of the stomach;

2 Branches of the nerve of Latarjet always run in a plane which is superficial to the vessels;

3 The nerves run for some distance along the walls of the stomach, adherent to the serosa, without branching, before penetrating the muscularis to innervate the mucosal syncitium.

56

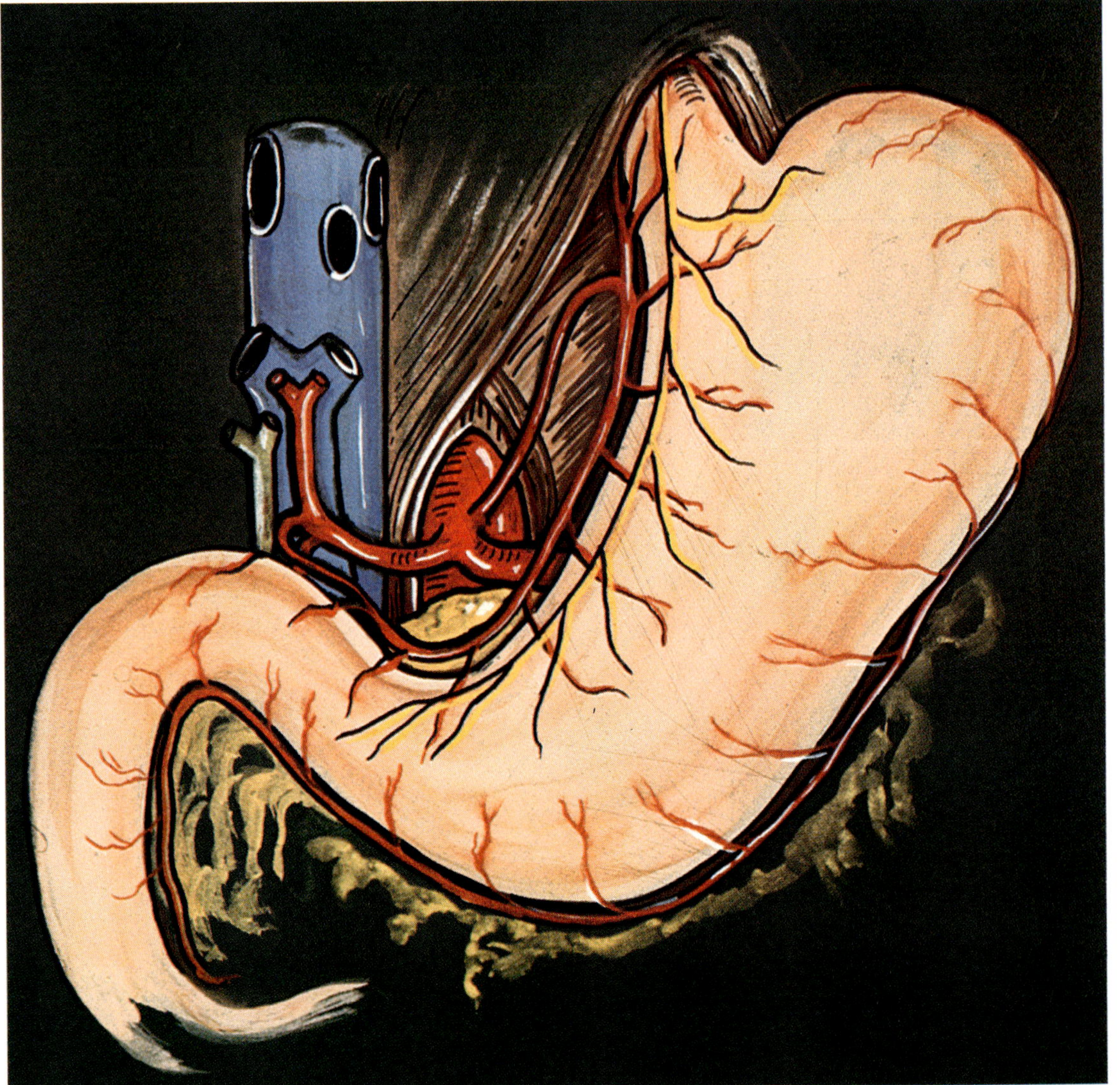

Seromyotomy begun

57 The nerve of Latarjet can be seen running along the lesser curve of the stomach; it often bifurcates, or even trifurcates quite high along the lesser curvature.

58 The seromyotomy is begun between 5 cm and 6 cm from the pylorus at the crow's foot. Two terminal branches of the nerve of Latarjet can usually be seen running onto the antral wall.

59 Branches of the nerve of Latarjet can here be seen running onto the anterior gastric wall at the incisura.

57

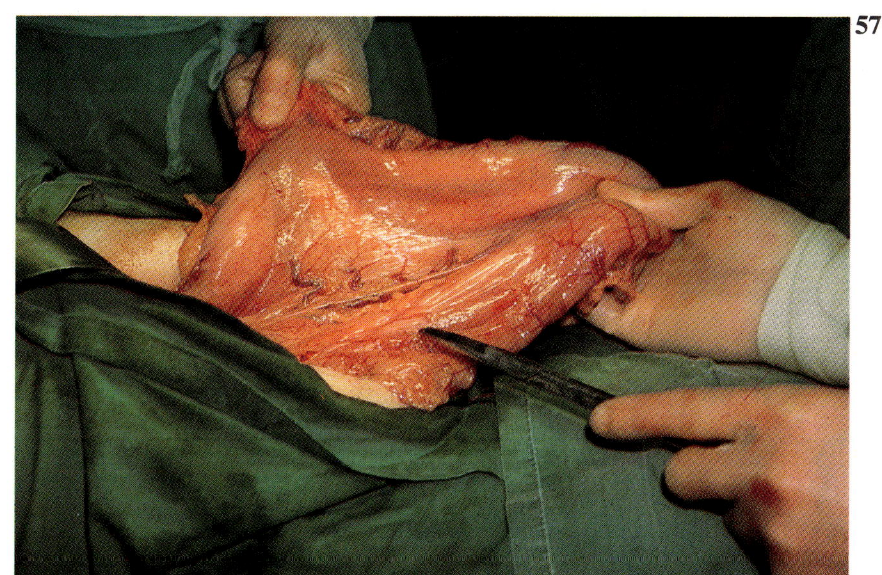

58

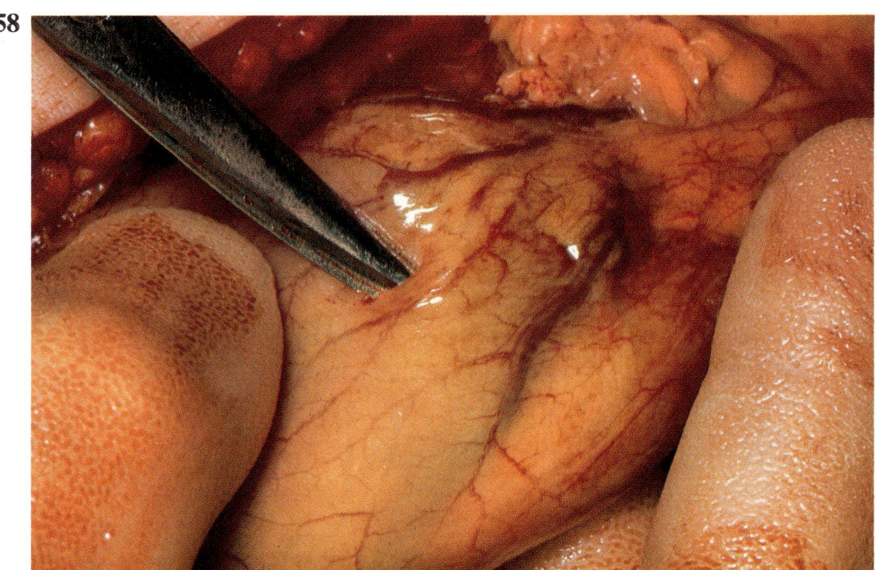

59

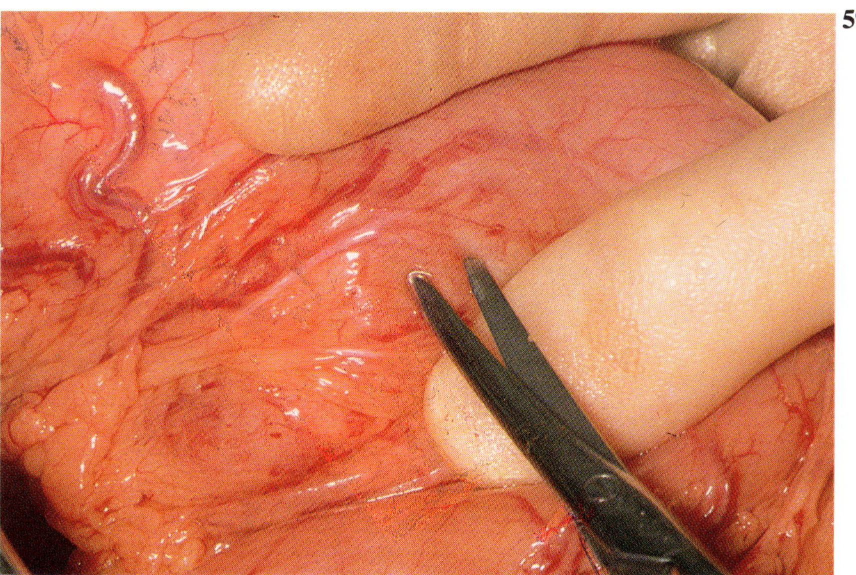

60 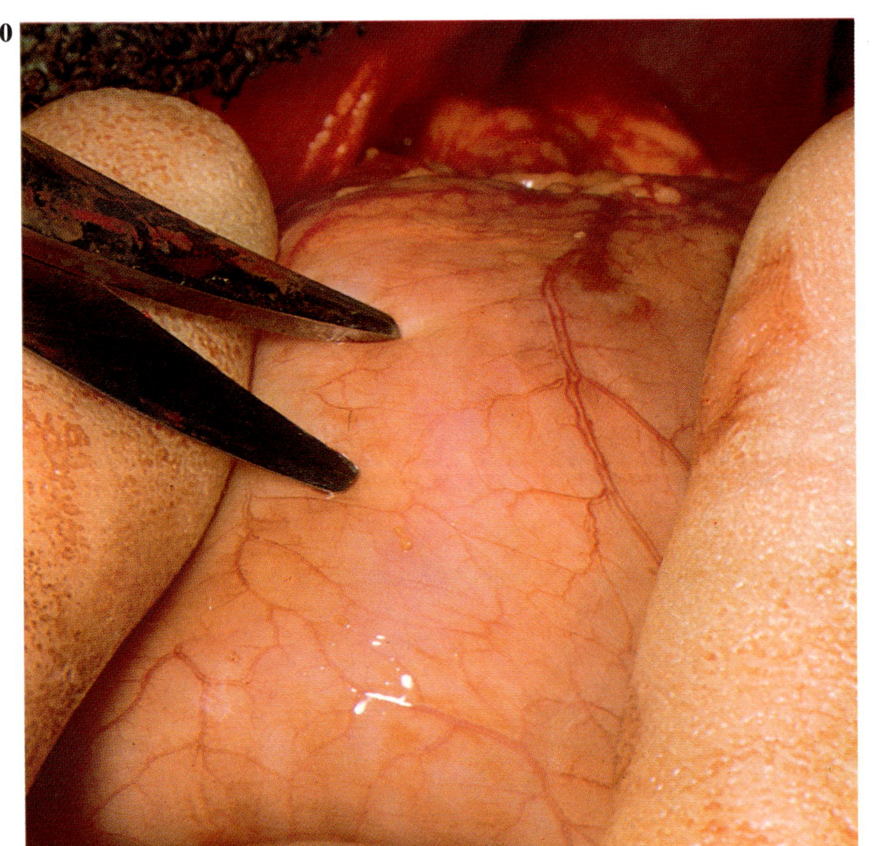

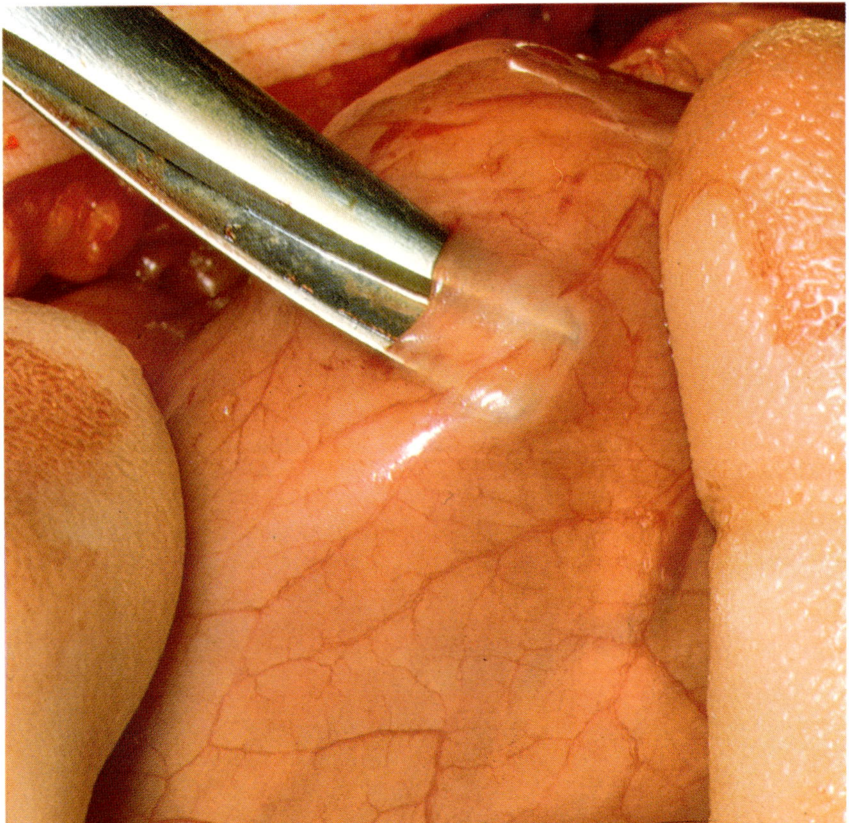 61

60 and 61 A point is chosen between 1.5 cm and 2 cm from the edge of the lesser curvature. Using blunt-nose scissors, the seromuscular layer is incised and the tips of the scissors are insinuated beneath the circular muscle layer.

Submucosal layer exposed

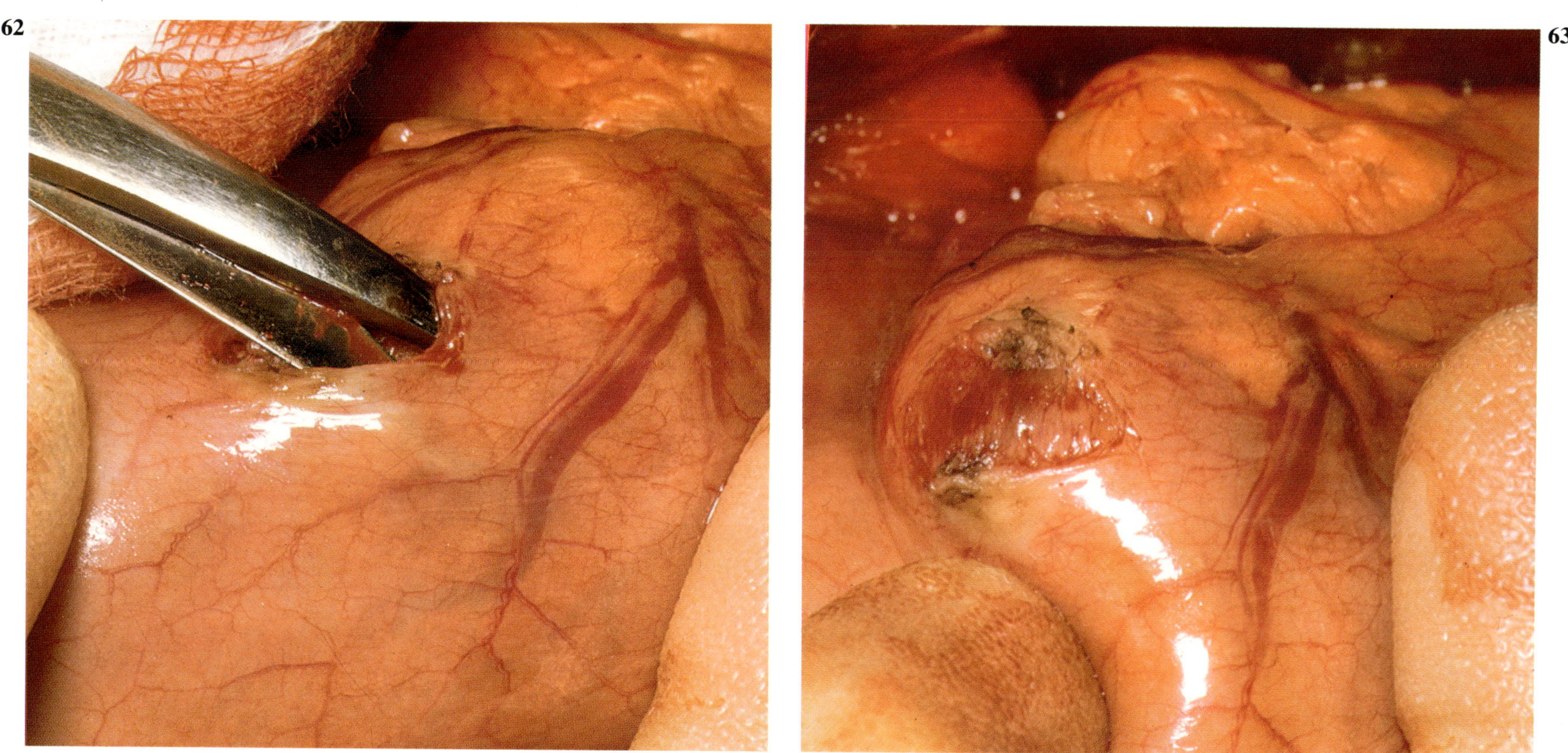

62 and 63 The submucosal plane is exposed.

64

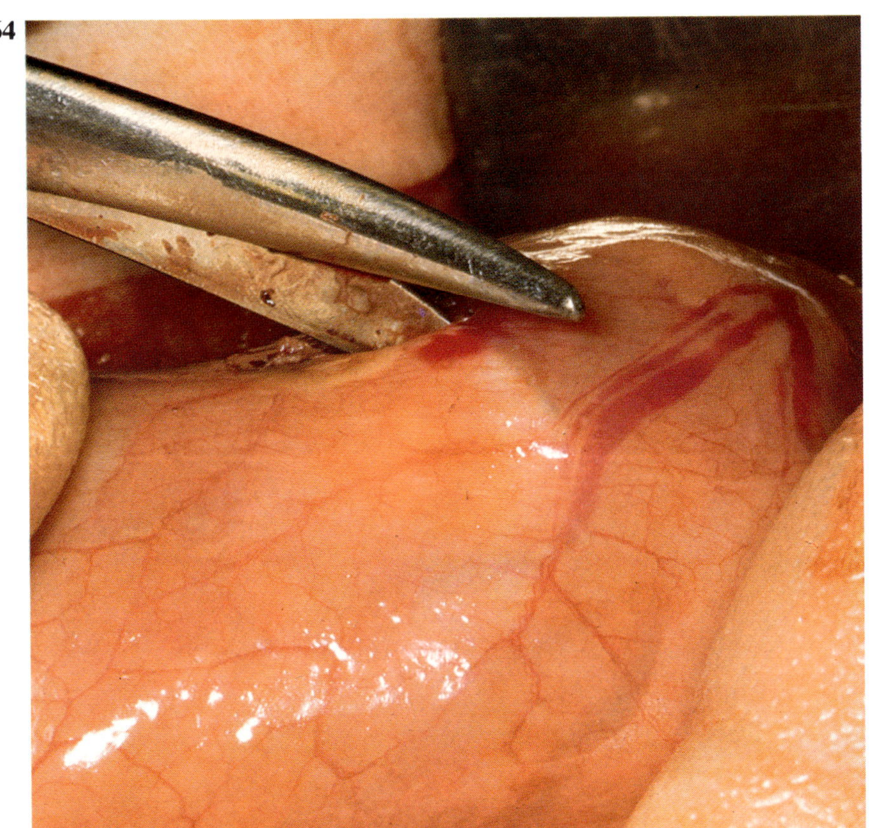

65

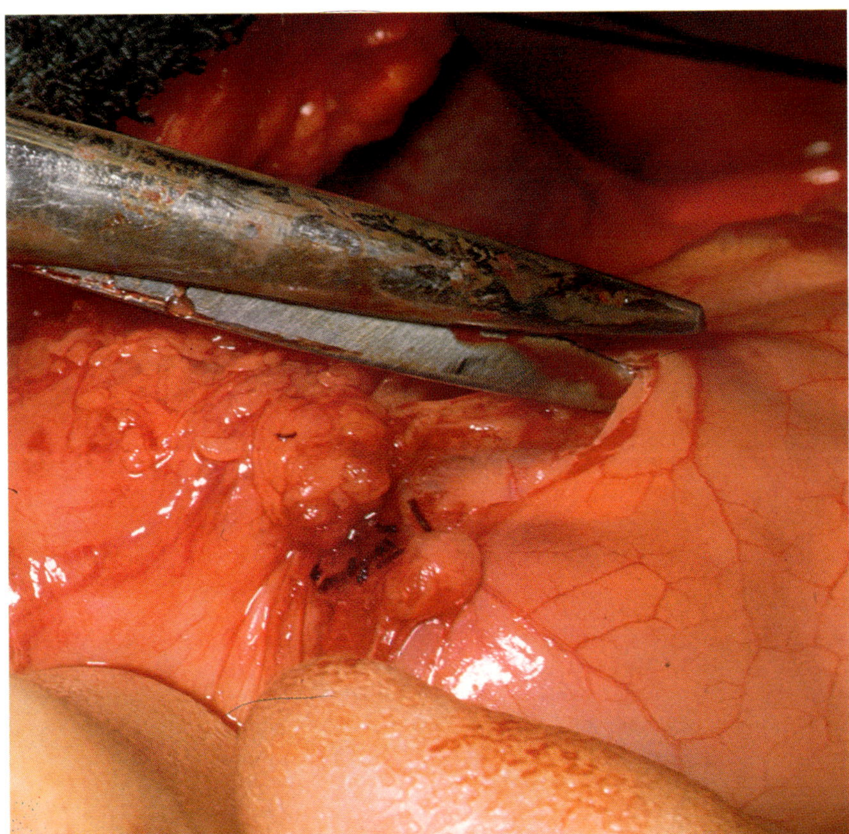

64 and 65 The seromuscular layer is next incised up to the first main leash of blood vessels, parallel to the lesser curvature and remaining about 1.5 cm from it.

66a

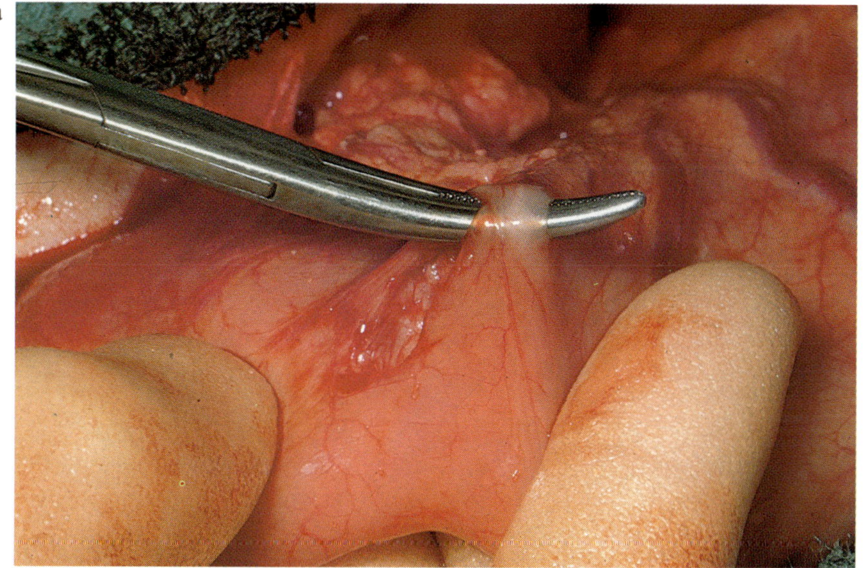

66b

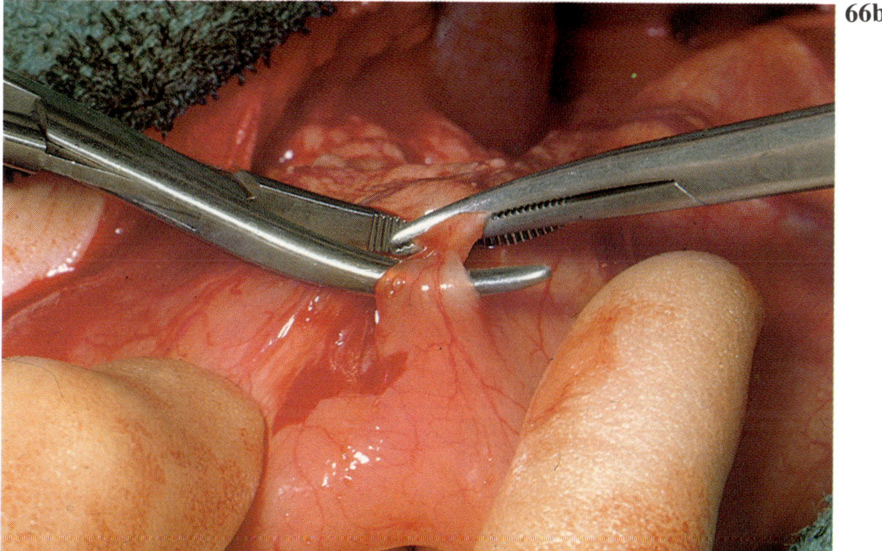

66 (a) A pair of Cairn's forceps is insinuated under the vascular bundle; (b) The vessels are clamped, divided – (c) and ligated.

66c

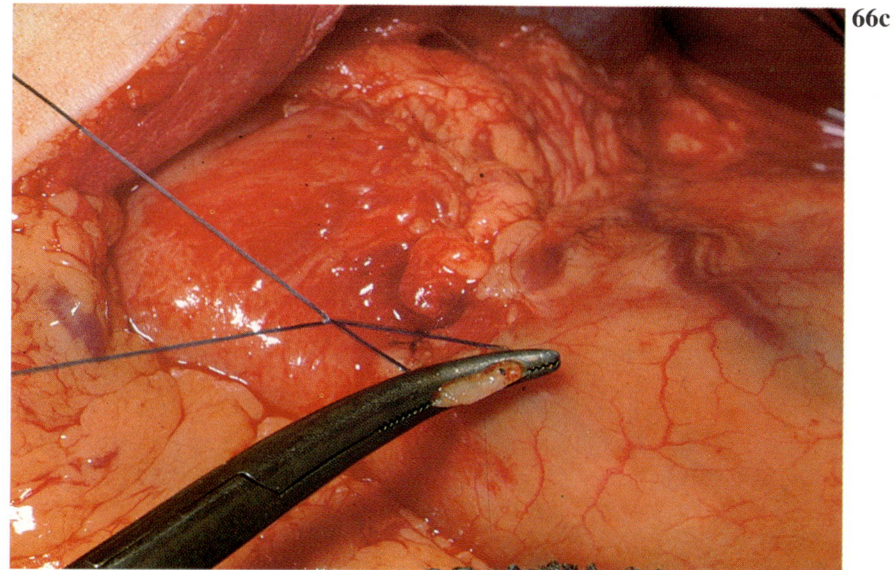

67

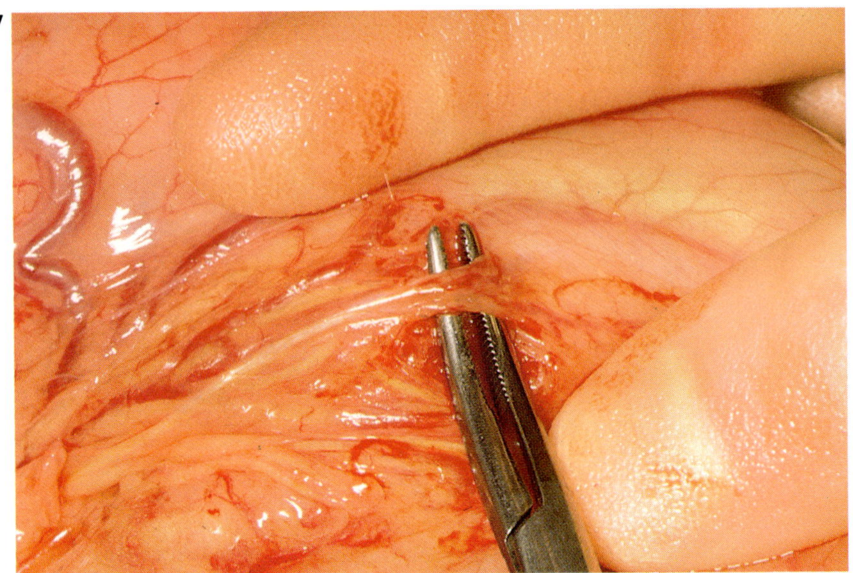

68

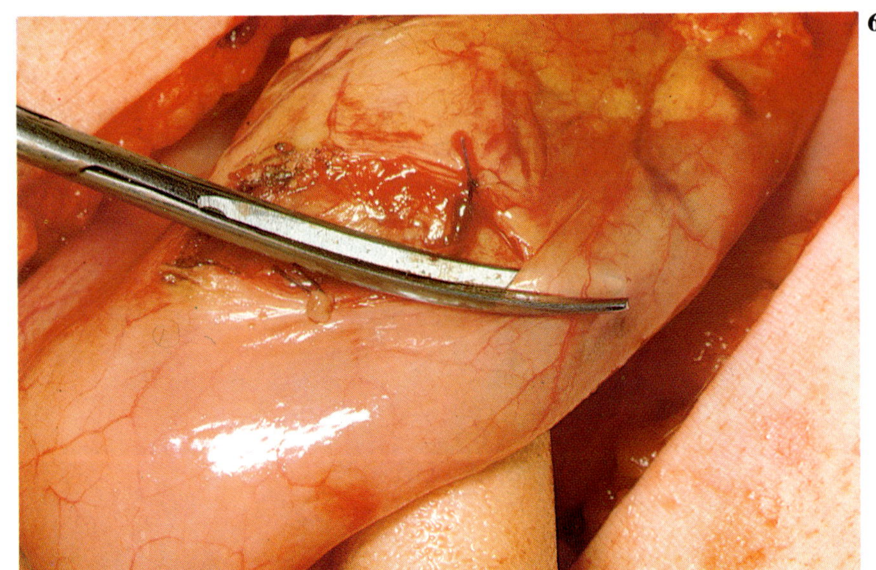

67 The plane of dissection can clearly be seen to be deep to the nerves and blood vessels.

68 and 69 The dissection is continued to the next vascular bundle exposing the submucosa beneath.

69

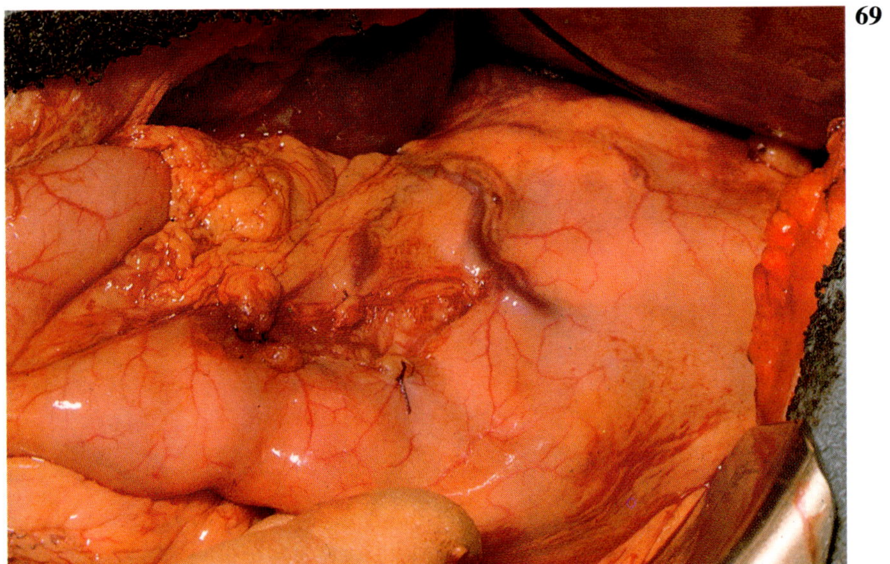

70
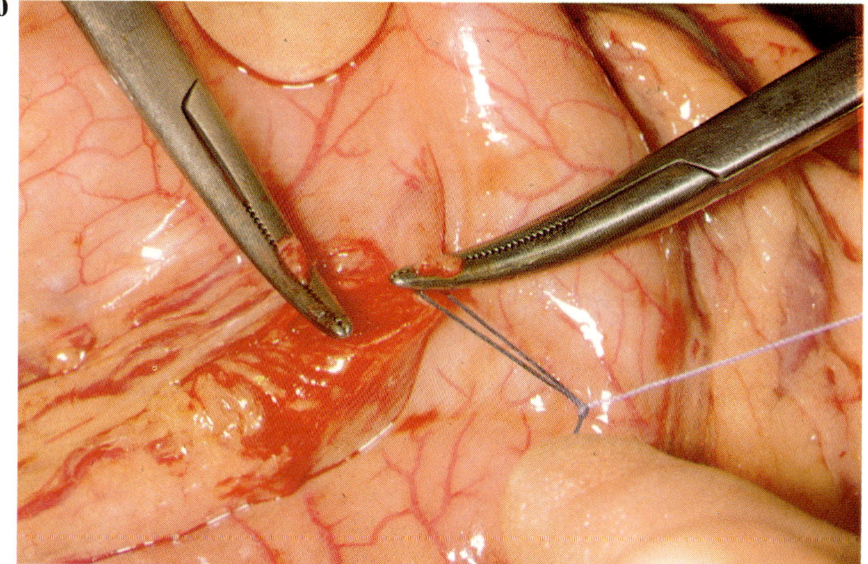

71
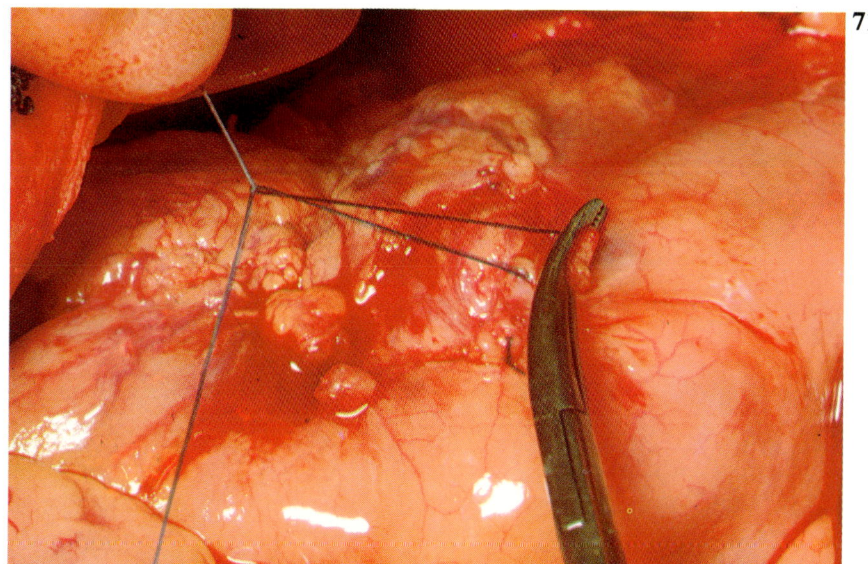

70 and 71 This next vascular bundle is divided and ligated.

72
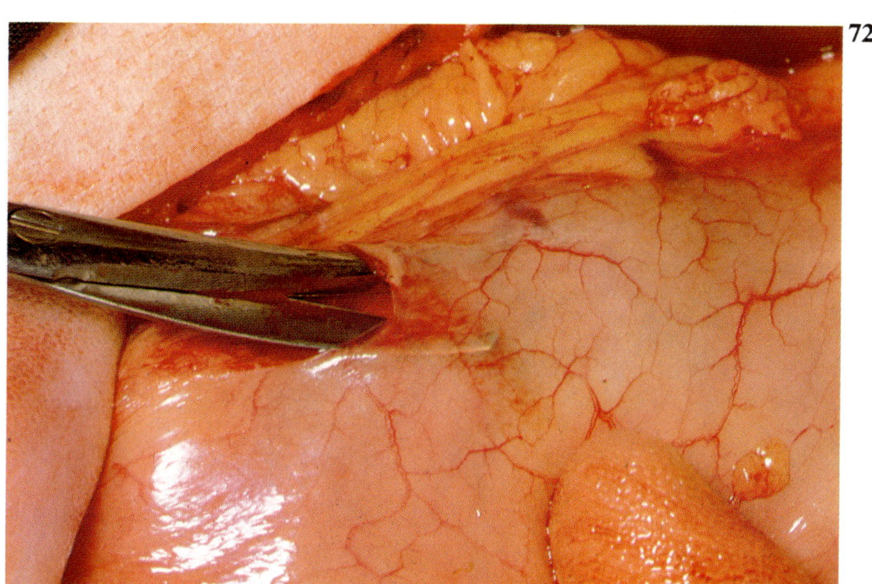

72 The dissection is further extended by insinuating the scissors deep to the seromuscular plane and spreading the tips of the instrument. Once in the correct plane, there is no difficulty in maintaining this as the seromuscular layers separate from the submucosa quite easily.

Further division of seromuscular plane

73

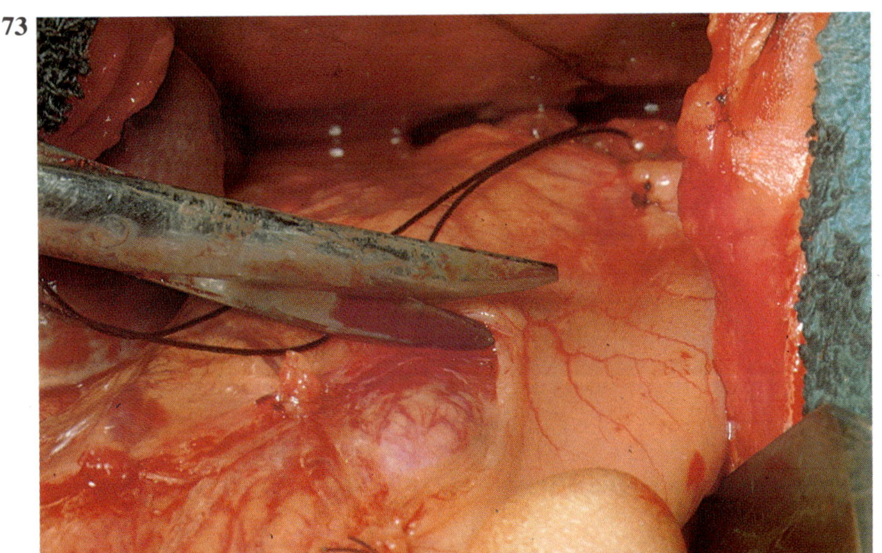

74

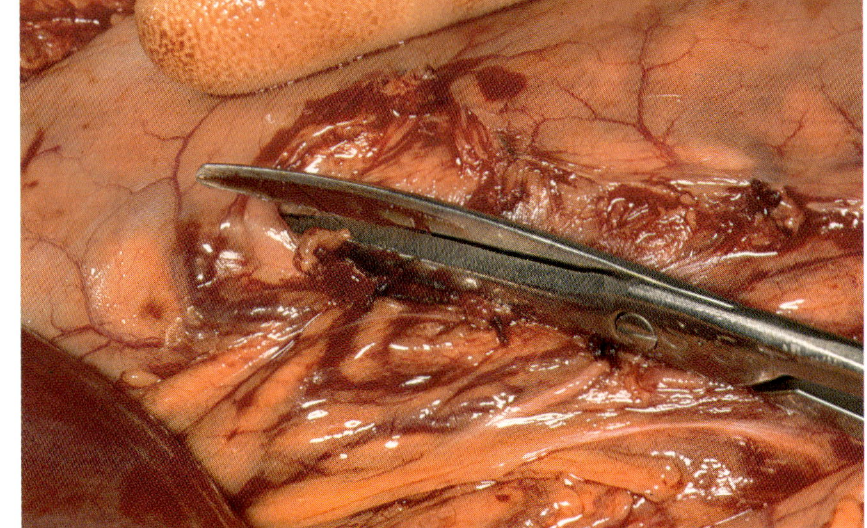

75

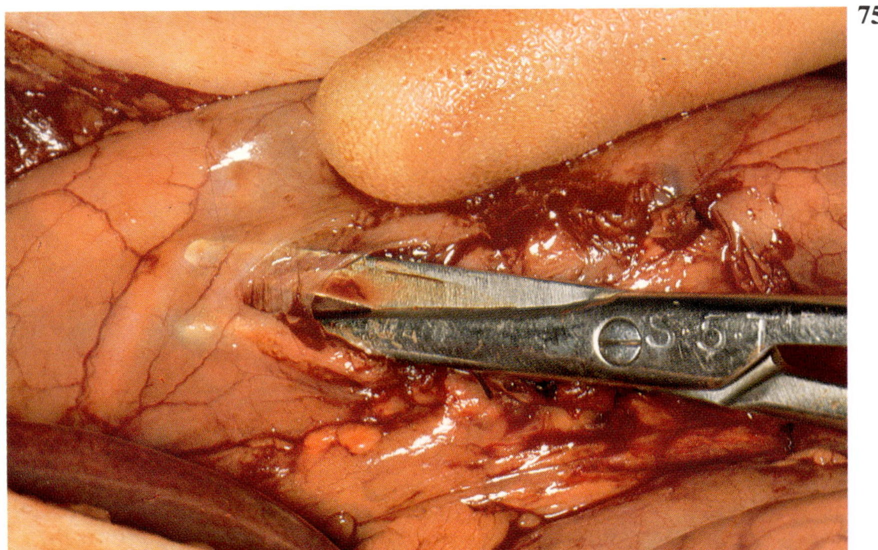

73 Further division of the seromuscular plane reveals the submucosa, which is exposed along the length of the myotomised segment.

74 The same technique is applied along the whole length of the lesser curvature: after division of a short segment –

75 – the scissors are spread gently beneath the next 1 cm to 2 cm of seromuscular tissue.

76

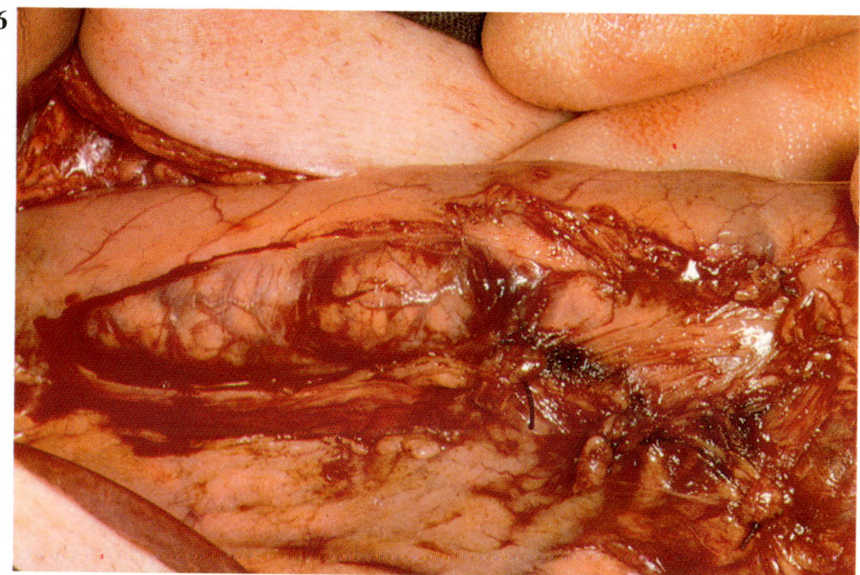

77

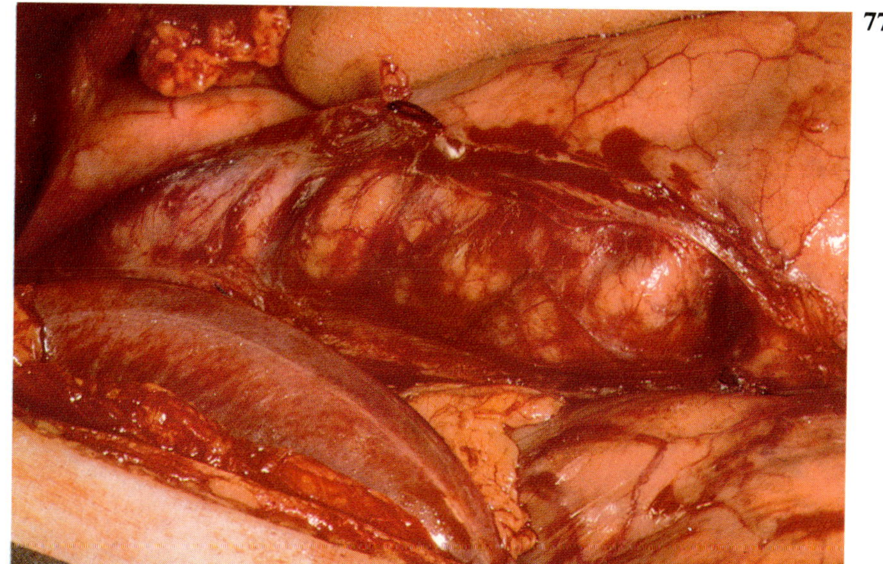

76 Quite wide separation of the divided seromuscular plane occurs exposing 1 cm to 2 cm of submucosa.

77 Few muscle fibres remain intact when using this technique. Of the three layers of muscle in the gastric wall, the outer longitudinal is inevitably divided with the middle and thicker circular layer. The innermost flimsy layer of oblique fibres is usually divided along with the circular muscle. If a few of these deep strands remain intact they need not be divided.

There is little or no risk of damaging the mucosa while using this technique. Should perforation occur, however, it is to be oversewn promptly with catgut and will later be protected by the overlap repair.

78 There are usually either three or four large vascular bundles between the crow's foot and the oesophagogastric junction which require ligating and dividing. The most proximal leash is often more conveniently clamped using Lahey forceps.

78

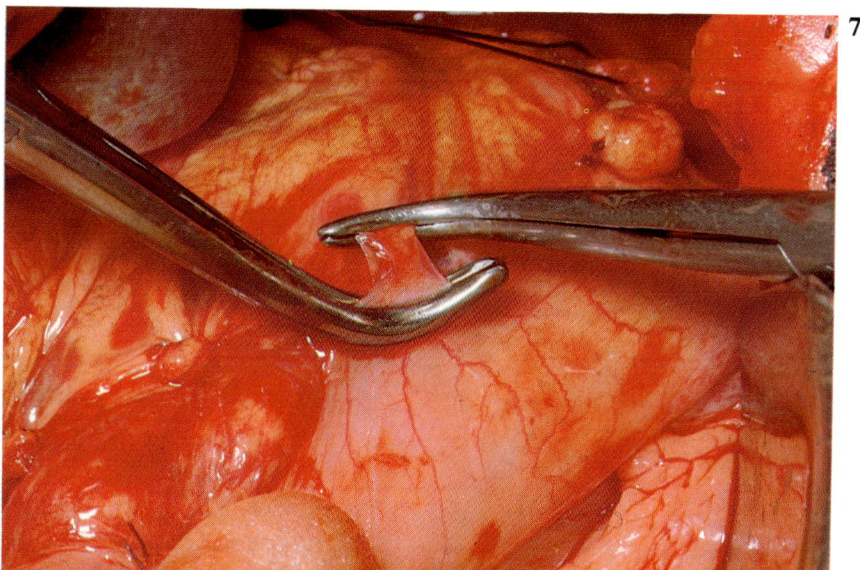

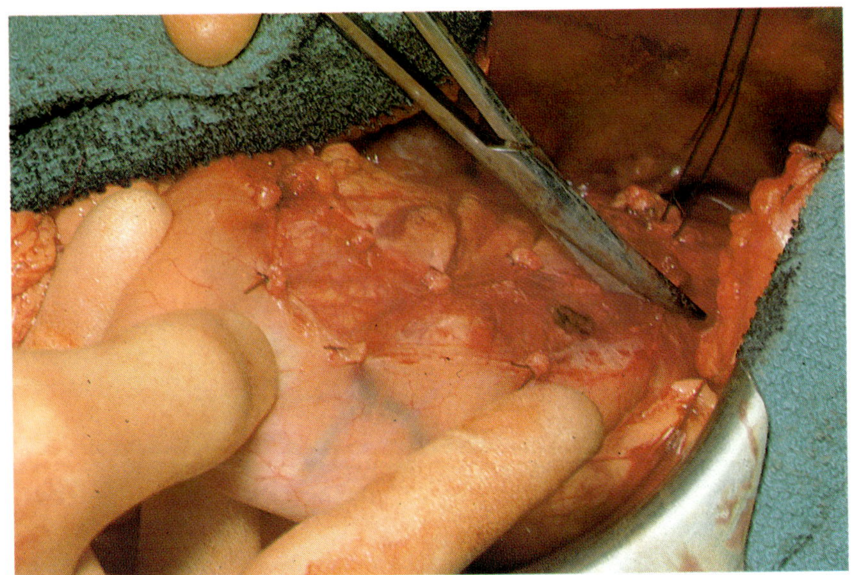

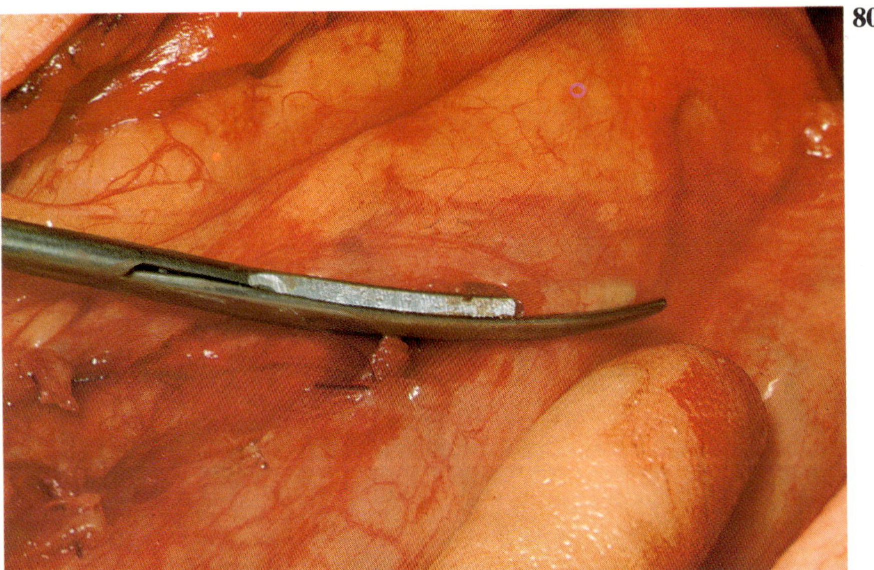

79 As the dissection extends more proximally the muscular layers become much thinner. The seromyotomy is completed at the level of the oesophagogastric junction.

80 The oesophagogastric junction is approached. The dissection stops at the top right of the picture at the point where the neurovascular bundle was divided (**40**); thus the lower oesophageal sphincter remains intact. Reflux oesophagitis has not been encountered after this procedure.

81 The completed proximal aspect of the seromyotomy is shown with the intact anterior vagus and the nerve of Latarjet lying well to the left of the line of dissection.

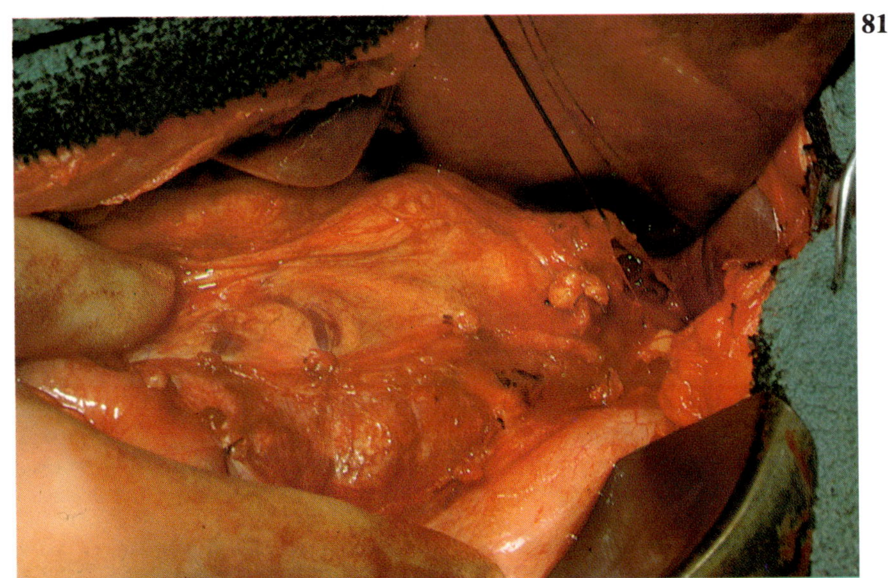

Overlap repair

82

83

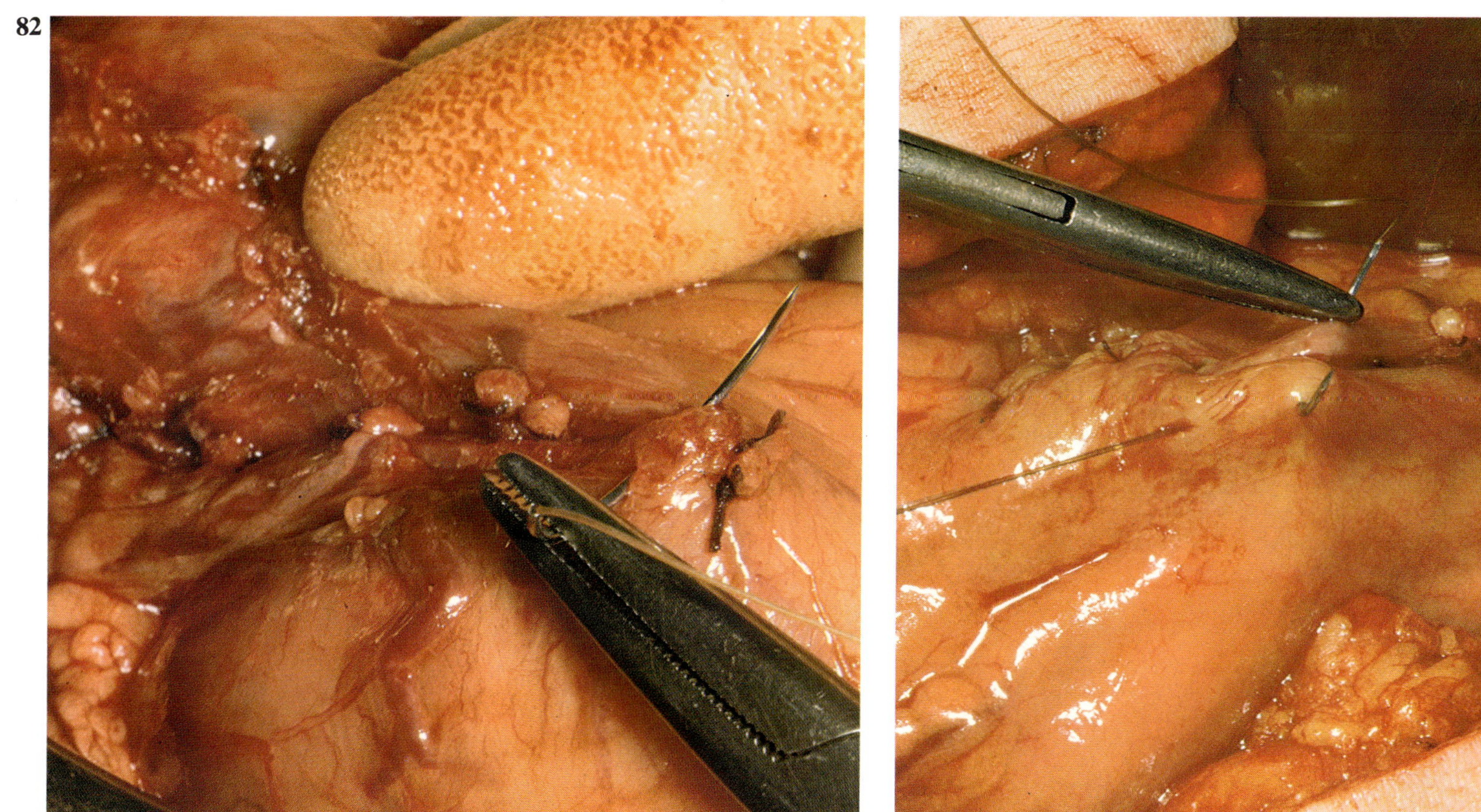

82 and 83 The serosal layer on the lesser curve aspect of the myotomised segment is next sutured over the defect, and across onto the serosa of the other side to begin an overlap repair.

84 The overlap repair is continued along the defect using a continuous catgut suture. The aim of the overlap repair is:

1 To reinforce the defect making any small risk of perforation less likely;

2 To prevent nerve sprouting into the underlying mucosa. (There is no evidence that sprouting nerve fibres can penetrate an intact serosa and underlying muscular layer.);

3 To prevent primary nerve regeneration between divided vagal nerve branches;

4 To reduce adhesion formation.

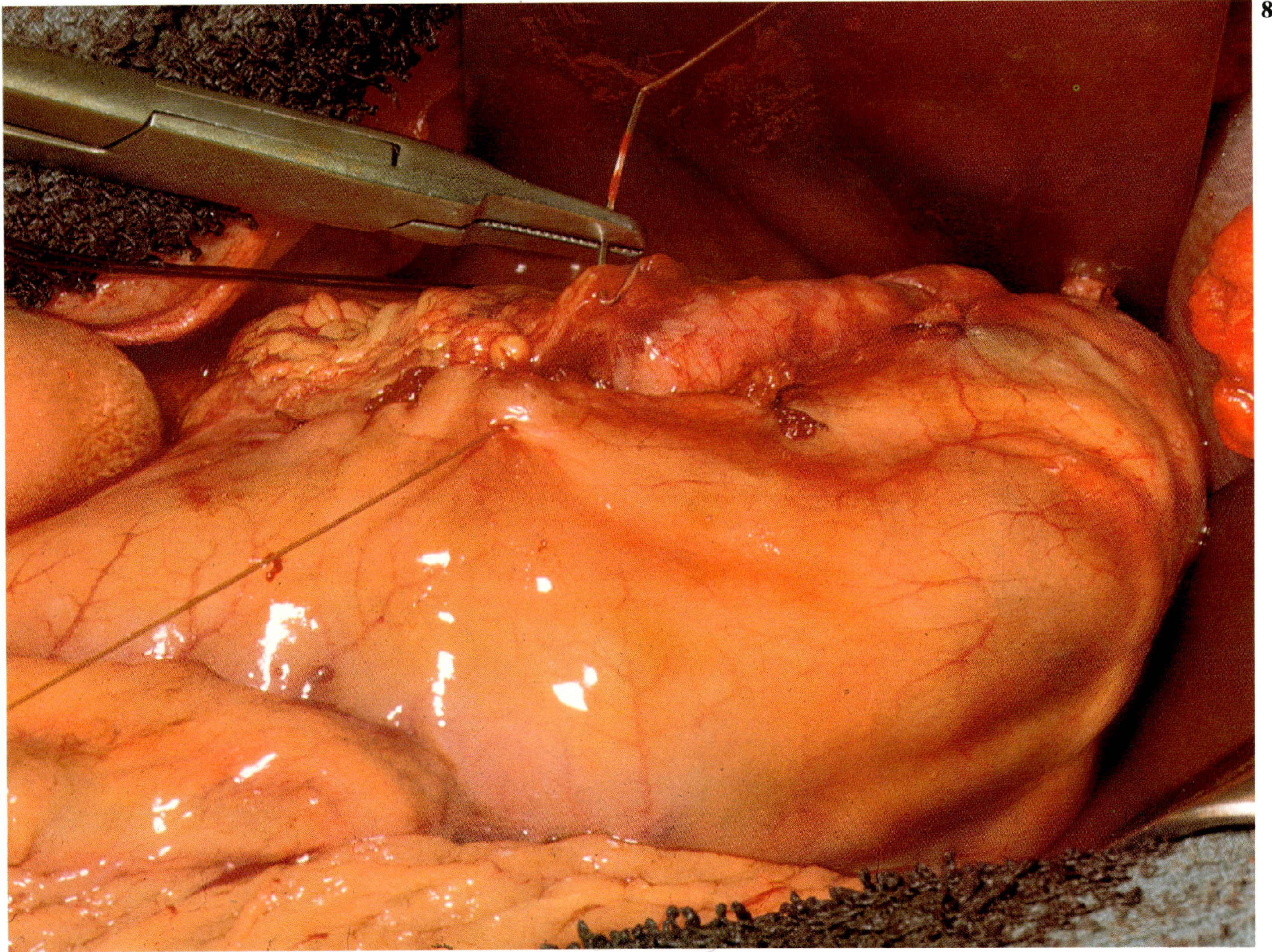
84

85 This repair is an overlapping of the sero-muscular layers and not a direct reanastomosis of the defect.

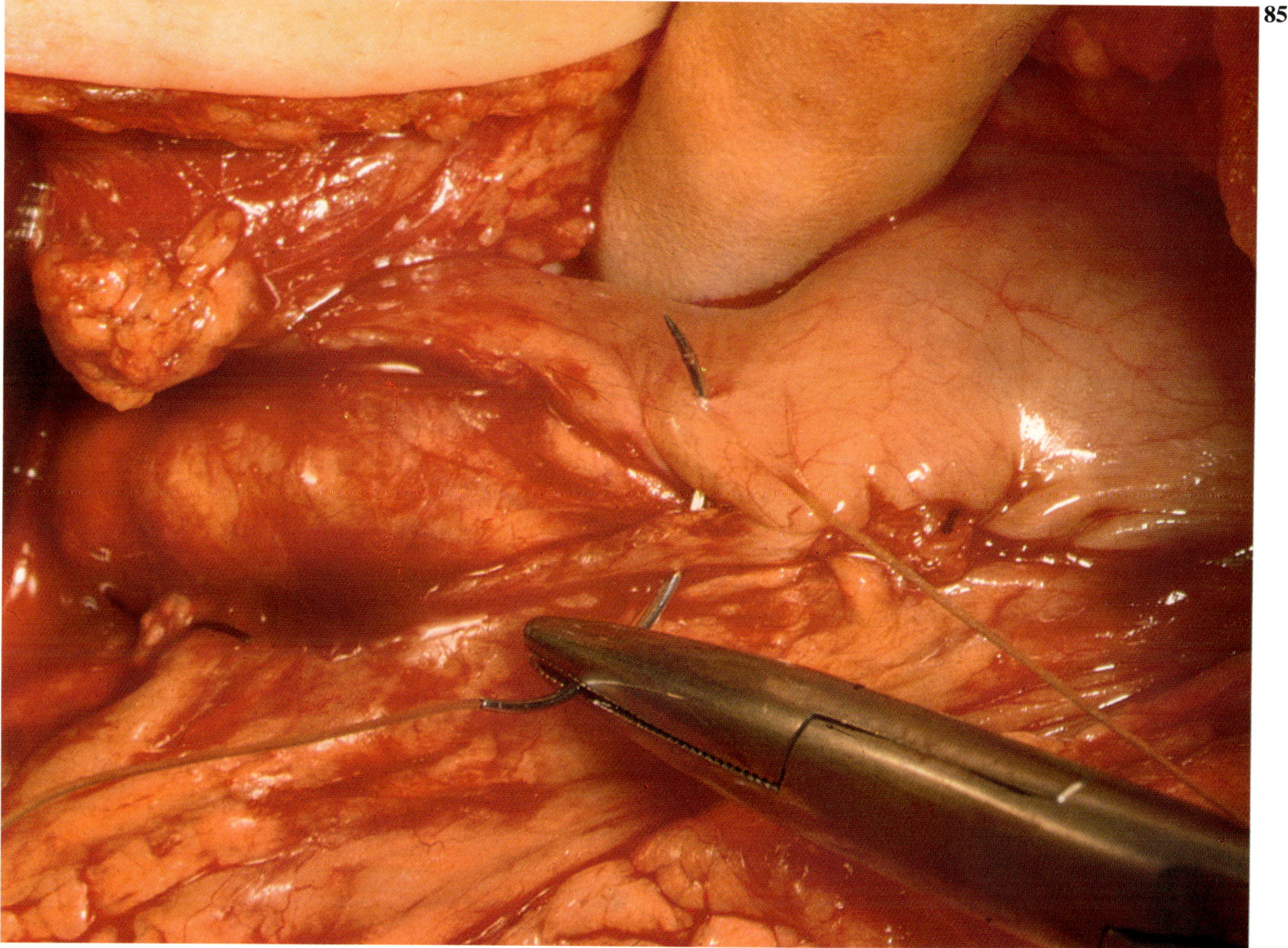

85

86 **The repair extends as far as the oesophago-gastric junction.**

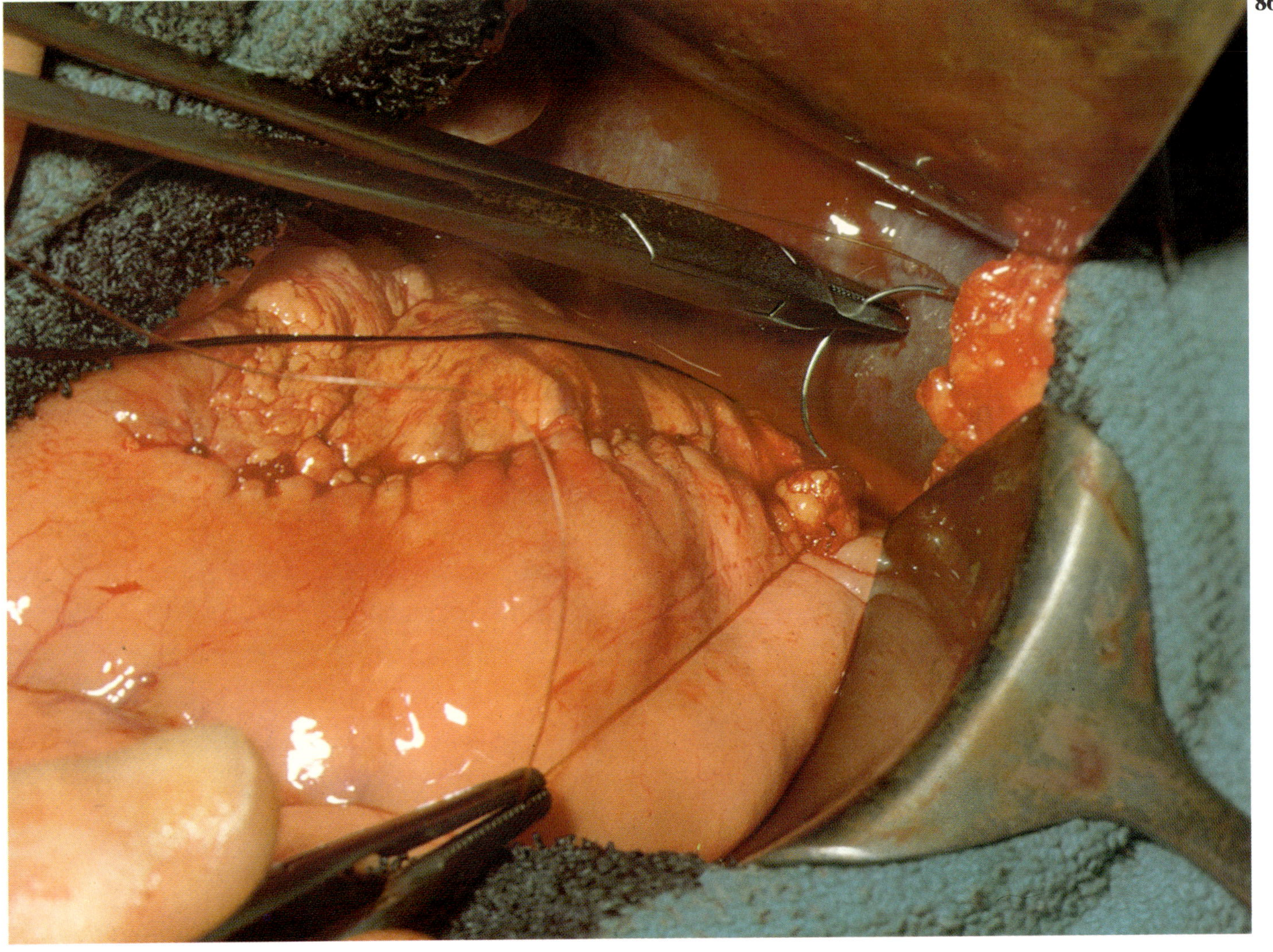

86

87 and 88 Differing views of the completed overlap repair. The stomach is pink and well perfused, there being no risk of ischaemic necrosis of the lesser curvature as the end arteries which directly enter the lesser curve remain intact.

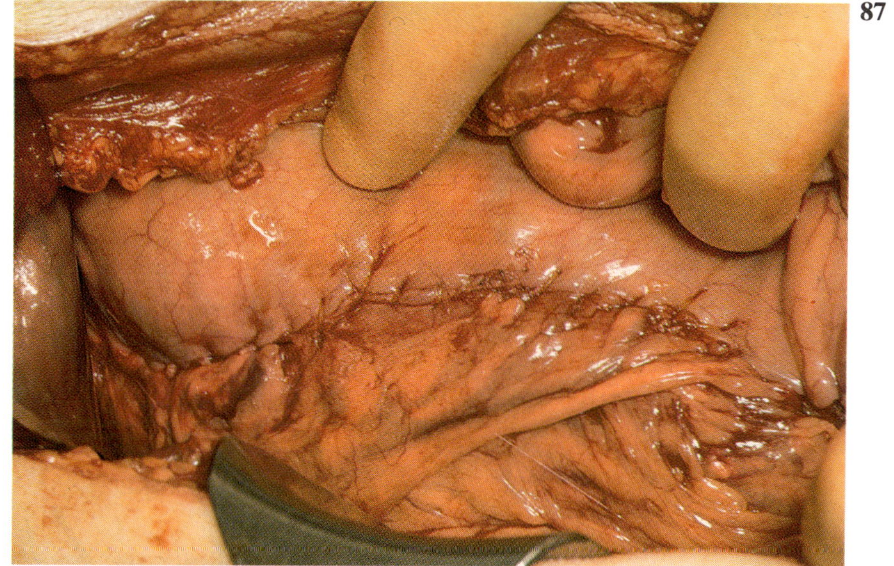
87

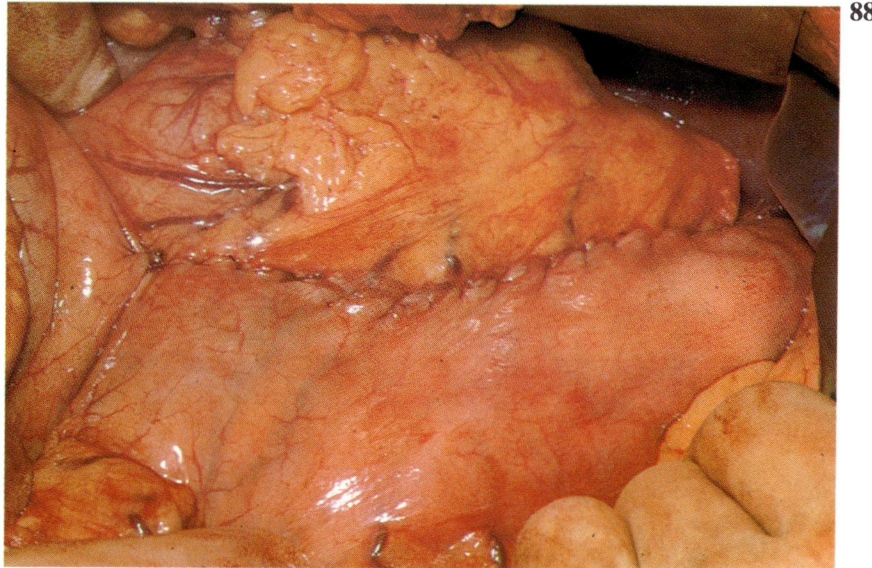
88

89 The intact anterior vagus nerve is here seen continuing as the nerve of Latarjet. There is no risk of damaging the anterior nerve of Latarjet in this operation, because it is well clear of the line of dissection. The integrity of this nerve is mandatory to transmit impulses to the antrum. Once the anterior antral wall is stimulated, intramural vagovagal arcs transmit the impulses through to the posterior wall of the antrum.

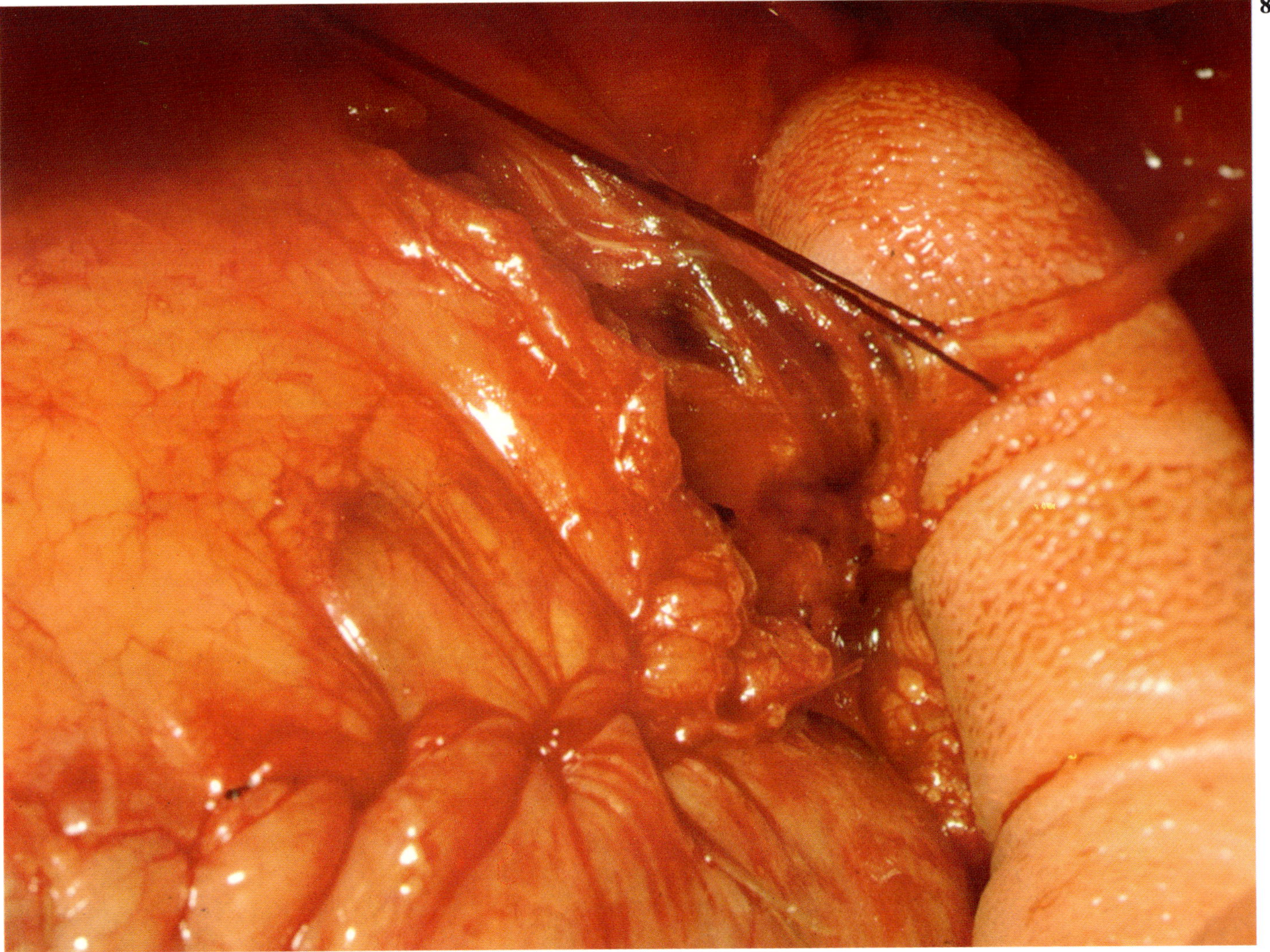
89

Preparation for closure of abdomen and its closure

90 Haemostasis is checked and the abdomen is prepared for closure. No drain is required.

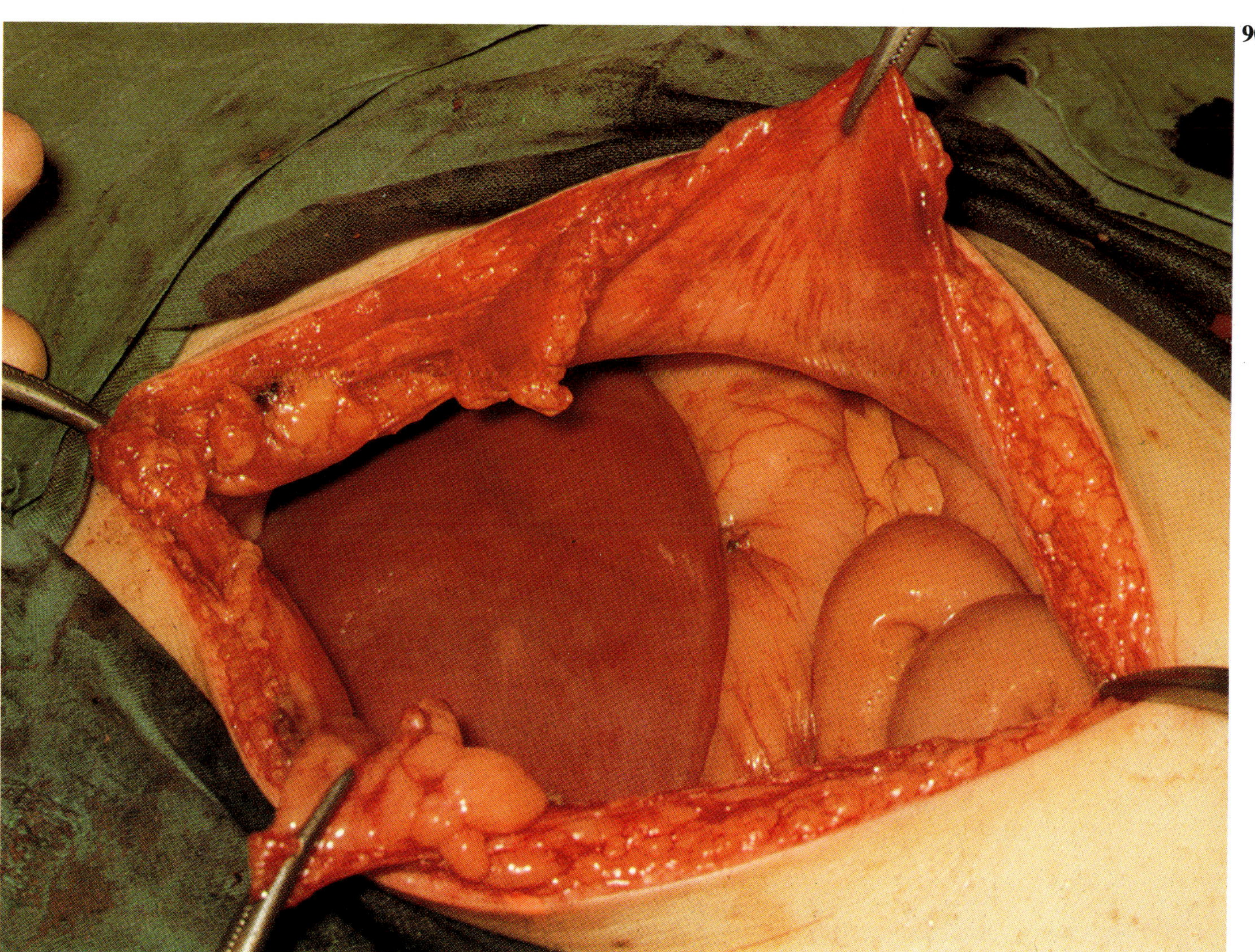
90

91 **The peritoneal layer is here being closed with a continuous layer of suture material.**

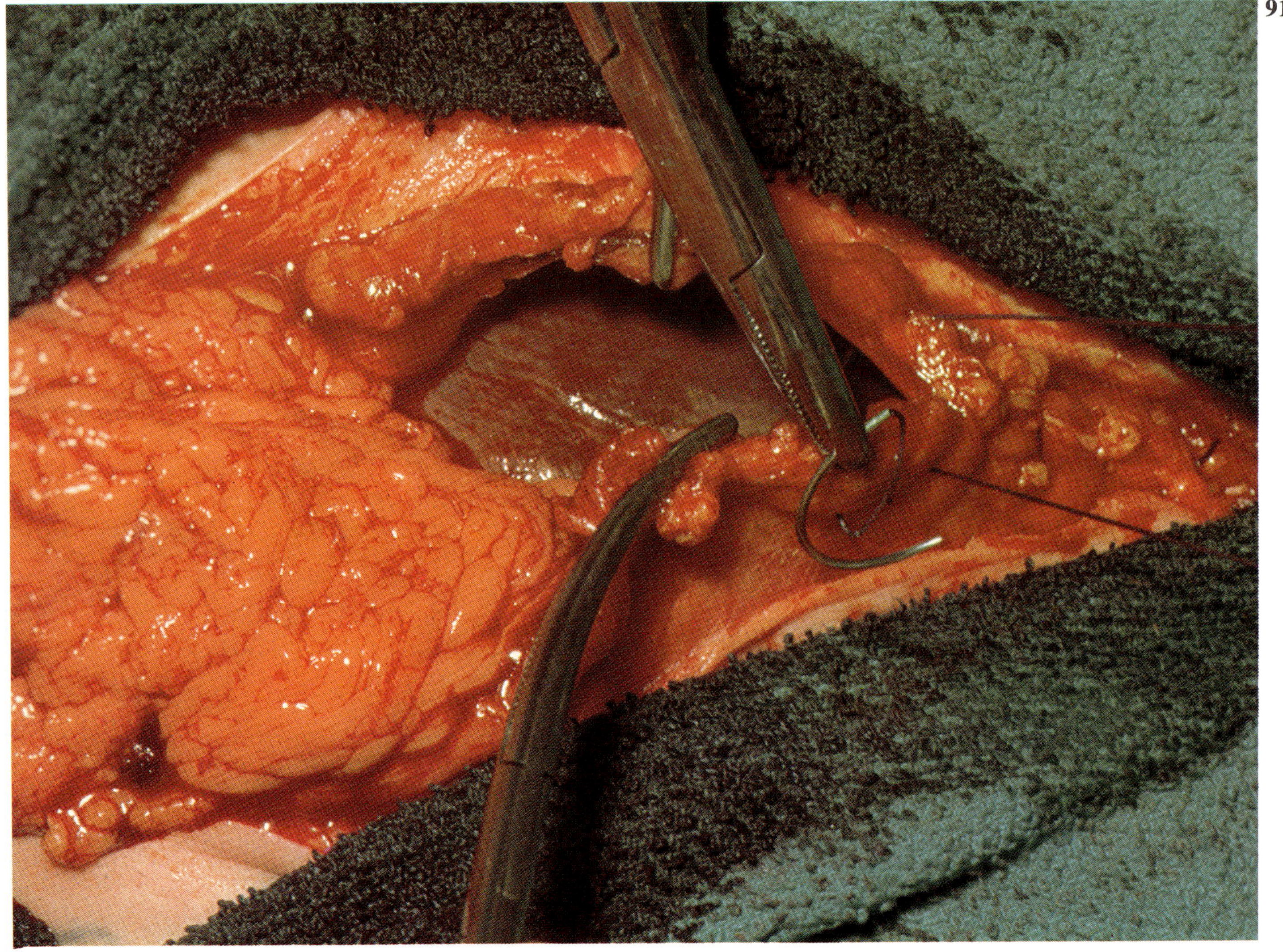

91

92 Closure of the peritoneum is complete.

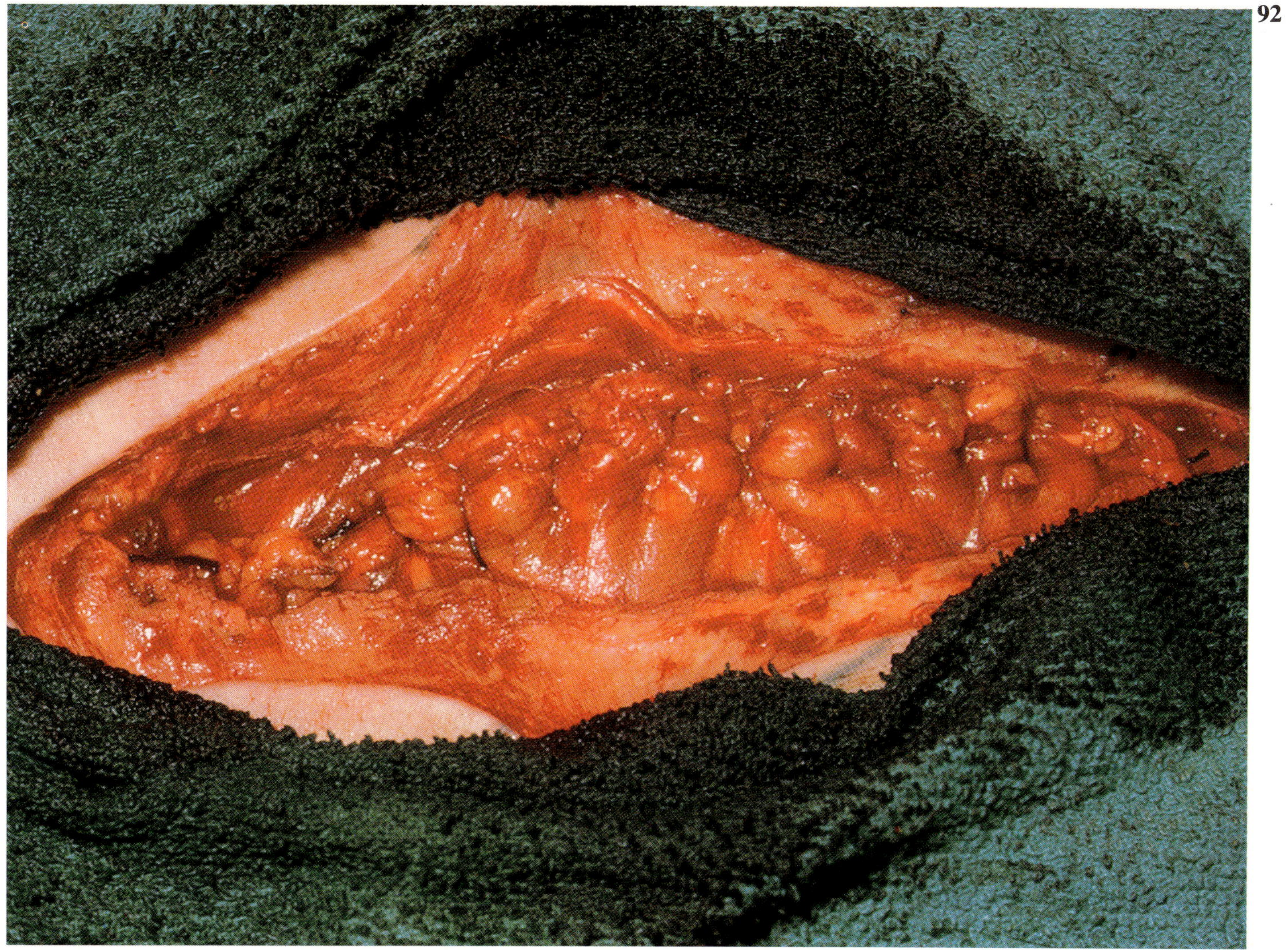
92

93 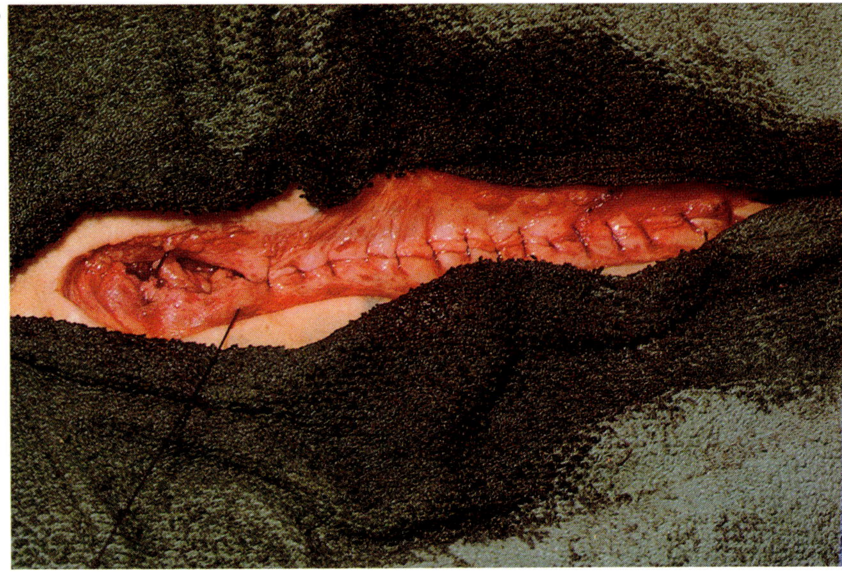

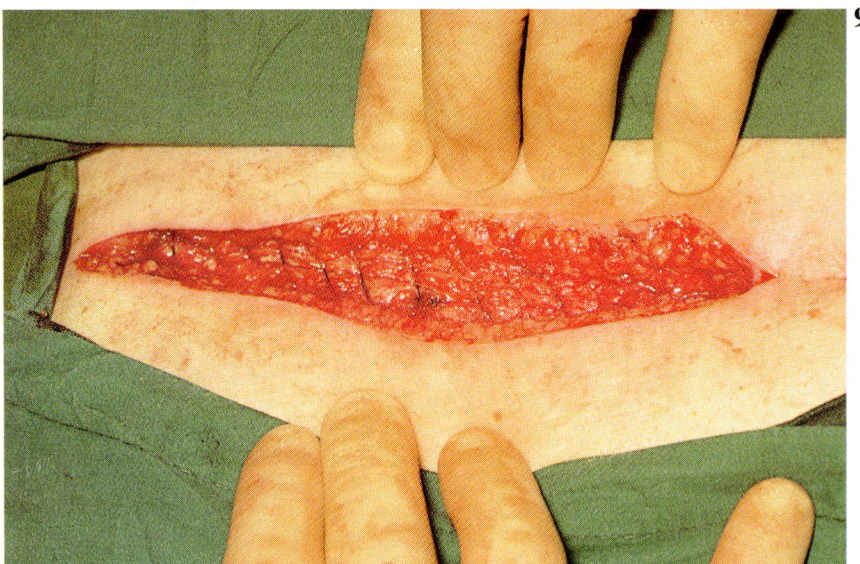 94

93 The linea alba is here being closed with a continuous suture.

94 The completed closure of the linea alba.

95 The skin has here been closed with a subcuticular suture.

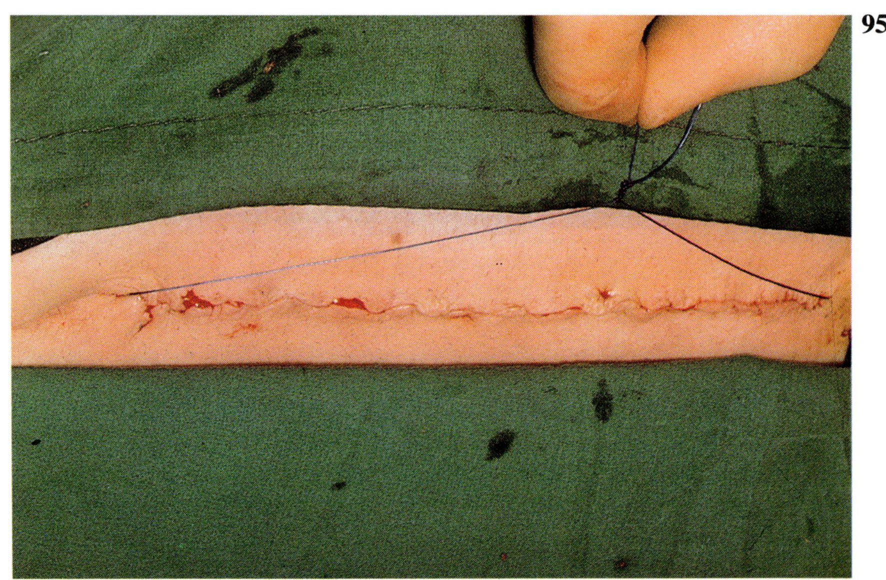 95

Conclusions

1 This operation is simple, safe and quickly performed.

2 Secretory studies have confirmed complete denervation of the parietal-cell mass.

3 Over 350 operations have been performed without a death.

4 Dumping and diarrhoea have been virtually abolished by preservation of the hepatic branches of the anterior vagus and the pylorus. When the above are preserved division of the posterior vagus trunk is not associated with postvagotomy sequelae. Occasional mild diarrhoea has been encountered in the early postoperative period, but so far has always resolved within three months.

5 Postoperative distension has not been marked, probably as a result of the myotomy which may compensate for the loss of adaptive relaxation of the stomach consequent upon vagotomy.

6 Preliminary results of a randomised controlled trial performed in Holland, in which this operation has been compared with conventional highly selective vagotomy, have shown that excellent results can be achieved with the seromyotomy operation. There was a greater degree of secretory inhibition after seromyotomy and the operating time was halved.

7 The operating time is similar to that in truncal vagotomy and pyloroplasty.

8 Gastric emptying is not delayed after this procedure; there is an increase in the early emptying of liquids but not of solids.

Index

All numbers refer to page numbers.

T

U

V

W

X